Sven-Olof Olsson

THE UNCONSCIOUS ZONE

The secret life of your brain

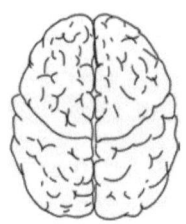

2016

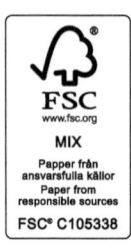

Förlag: BoD - Books on Demand, Stockholm, Sverige
Tryck: BoD - Books on Demand, Norderstedt, Tyskland
ISBN: 978-91-7699-220-3

Cover illustration: Illustration of the concepts of the
conscious, preconscious and unconscious according to
psychoanalysis theories of Sigmund Freud.

Content

Introduction
Intuition and the unconscious zone

The concept of "The Unconscious Zone" in this book pertains to our mind areas where many intuitive decisions and subliminal influences are unconsciously. As people are we exposed daily for hidden impacts that are not recorded by our consciousness. We says that we have decided after our gut feeling or that we, without conscious knowledge, intuitively just know how something is connected. Many famous scientists (for example Einstein, Maxwell) have shown to their intuition when they suddenly discover new previously unknown lows in physics. New findings in brain research on perception suggest that our consciousness only to a little extent can take advantage of all the information as our senses produce.

Brain researchers have shown that we have a delay of approximately 0.5 seconds before we become aware of such as sights that are generated in order of 10 MB/s (10 million bits of information per second). This delay would be able to be fatal in situations where we need to react instinctively when any dangerous occurrence (escape, risk of injury). The brain has solved this by reacting automatically without a conscious mind in many situations. If we for example run the car   often do not know how we have operated the car forward to destination, then driving has become an automatic activity until it eventually something happens unexpectedly.

We may in many cases work out a capability to automatically conduct as a Budo sports, in which the body is trained to instinctively perform appropriate parades without conscious intervention. Even in many monotonous work situations tend we perform work to daydreaming, while the body automatically performs the learned work phases. As difference from previous position is

"Flow" a special condition where you go into a task and literally engulfed by the workflow and to become unaware of time and environment. It requires some prerequisites for that end up in the flow State.

We are also talking about hidden (silent) knowledge in different work areas, which sometimes says that the company's knowledge is sitting in the walls. Faithful employees with many years of experience in a company have often an unconscious knowledge which, as it was, sitting in the spinal cord. An example is from Ericsson Microwave (former employment) where a waveguide for microwaves to Tele-X satellite with especially high demands on accuracy (1/100 mm) were turned. They got hire a pension based turners with long experience of a special lathe in order to keep the necessary accuracy of the wave guide.

In everyday life is contemporary man prone to unconscious influences in many contexts. Behavioral Science has revealed our buying habits and thus designed the stores to merchandising, the lighting, the color and background music has been adapted in order to trigger optimal needful things of the customer. Even the advertising industry is exploring how best to get the attention of newspaper ads and TV commercials. In this context, talking man of subliminal perception where we have made attempts to put in the occasional advertising images in movies which we do not see consciously but that nevertheless can give subconscious message.

A different unconscious influences which we daily suffer for is our relationship to body language. We have more often an intuitive way to interpret the signals as the surroundings gives. Chapter 6 provides an overview of how we can become aware of this influence.

New development of electronic devices for measurement via electrodes on the body by normal unconscious endocrine functions has resulted in a new therapy work activities referred to as biofeedback. The equipment is designed so that the patient visually or sonically can see the current status of the measured variable. Through biofeedback can you affect the heart rate with conscious suggestions and immediately see the effects on pulse rhythm. Therapeutic biofeedback is used to, among other things affect stress-related medical conditions. Similar effects on the body's endocrine system, it has in thousands of years been able to influence via Yoga training. Methods for reducing the respiratory rate, heart rate and metabolism are included in many Yoga traditions.

Later time brain research has completely new possibilities to measure the brain's internal work by identifying the neural networks via computer-controlled measurement methods such as functional magnetic resonance tomography (fMRI) and Magnetoencephalography (MEG) and Transcranial magnetic stimulation (TMS) and others. Through these methods can we today in detail follow the brain's work and identify many of the unconscious activities that shape our thoughts. For people with neurological disorders, this will result in completely new treatments.

Hypnosis is used in medicine as stunning at certain operations, and as therapy for, among other things smoking cessation and curative of phobia. More recent research has shown that hypnosis is a special State of consciousness in which to measure eye movements and EEG (measuring electrical activity in the brain via electrodes on the outside of the scalp) which gives specific patterns that differ from normal awake consciousness.

Placebo/nocebo effects that affect us, among other things in disease treatment have been identified via modern research methods. Even in Sweden carried out this type of research at the Karolinska hospital in Stockholm under the leadership of Professor Martin Ingvar. Results from the placebo research have already had an impact on the development and testing of new medicinal preparations to safeguard the positive impact that placebo can bring.

In psychoanalytic terms, according to Freud, so he talks about different layers in the personal consciousness that he resembles at the iceberg which floats on the water's surface. Over the surface of the water is the conscious ego and beneath the surface is the subconscious as similar to iceberg have the greatest content. Water surface is symbolized by the term preconscious containing perception which can be reached with some effort.

C G Jung, one of Simon Freud's earlier assistant, drew up its own theory when he introduced the term the collective unconscious state where the concept of archetypes was introduced.

In the book outlines for parts of the latest research results of the brain's complex neurological structure. In Chapter 3 "Can brain be hacked" is given a selection of brain research that in a future even that can penetrate below the skull and register the inner monologue of an experiment object. Chapters in the book can be read independently of each other as articles in each topic area. Each chapter ends with a summary of its contents. Chapters 1 and 2 provide a more neurological background regarding the brain's inner workings. Tentatively, it is in the table of contents, select any chapter that arouses most interest to read first and then read about the neurological background in chapters 1 and 2. Then each chapter keep new definitions and background descriptions should be in order to get a full understanding of the book "The Unconscious Zone" do a second reading from the beginning to what is between the lines shall be shown.

Chapter 1 Consciousness, human's perception and limitations

The universe of neurons

The human brain as well as the deep seas is two of the planet's remaining non-researched white places, where the science stands before big challenges. Mankind has relatively recently invented tools for being able to identify the physiological-strategic processes in the brain witch humanity earlier only have been able to explore through speculation and assumptions. During the last few decades in the context of the fast computer development have brain researchers got new methods of magnetic imaging (fMRI), EEG, PET, MEG and TMS. These methods have open possibility's to map out the many different activities in the brain's neural networks and led to that we started to make out individual thoughts in a person's brain. The human brain is probably the most complicated structure in the universe with about 100 billion brain cells (neurons) and where each neuron can have up to 10000 nerve connections with other neurons in the gigantic network. The complexity of these networks carrying gigantic amount of connections and in comparison are current supercomputers, far from being able to simulate these complex neural networks.

Researchers have successfully mapped the genetic information in the human genome within an international project for 10 years on the project, HUGO (Human Genome Organization). Recently started a long-lasting project in the United States at UCLA University in Los Angeles where the research under the direction of Professor in Neurology, Arthur Toga on corresponding way should identify the entire brain neural network. This project is called "The human connectome project". In Europe there is a similar 10-year project entitled "Human Brain Project" (HBP), which focuses on with computer simulation of single neural network gradually try to make simulation of the whole brain networks.

It is said often that we as humans use only about 10 % of our brain power. The truth is probably in the reverse that the majority of the processes in brain, about 90 %, are unconscious, while we are conscious of approximately 10%. The brain can be compared to today's computers, which now used parallel computing cores that can process data at the same time to increase computational performance. Similarly handles brain stimuli from our minds in different parallel neuron network which gives a tremendous increased data processing and simultaneous capacity.

The book's title "The Unconscious Zone" would try to give an understanding of all the unconscious processes that are going on in our brain. In the following Chapters describes many of the things that are going on in our brains there we typically are unaware of its impact on our emotions, behaviors and decisions. In this first chapter gives more general properties of the human brain to be described in order to provide background information regarding basic anatomy, physiology and cognitive properties. If the reader wants to immerse themselves in some of these special topics there are given suggestions to literature in the book's reference list. The heading of this chapter "the universe of neurons" would point to the importance of the neurons various network whose complexity is comparable with our current knowledge of the universe's unimaginable size.

Despite that we in our conscious mind as a human experiencing the world as a tridimensional continuous experience (analog), there are many limitations in our senses and in the brain's processing of the incoming stimuli from our surroundings. Our sense of time can for example be affected partly by the emotional content where a certain dull activity can give a perpetual long boring feeling. While the experience of time in childhood, when the most experience is new, due to a summer holiday can be experienced as an eon of time. But in adult age you think that the vacation in the summer just goes too fast. Purely philosophical one can consider what is meant by time and how the causal event processes together in terms of present, future and past (history).

One who pondered deep in these matters is a church father Augustine of Hippo (years 354-430) who in his classic book "Confessions" (book 11, § 17-41, ref. 1.1) in connection with thoughts about how God created the world, gave his views on how we as humans experience time. Augustine notes like Aristotle: that all know what time is, until they will be asked what time is. Augustine's indicates that time is related to events in the past (past tense), things that is ongoing (present) and things that are expected to be in the future. Already there notes Augustine an obvious thing, if time is defined by things that will happen, persist for a short period of time and then disappear the time as an ultimate consequence is undefinable. When Augustine asks the question of how far the present is: year, months, one day, one hour, one minute or one second, he comes to the conclusion that the present moment is only the transition between future and past and thus do not have a degree, but only the line in between. He notes that the present time not taking any space and has no extent, then each duration would instantly become past and future yet not exist. The past (past tense) are not existing but survives as the pictures in the memory in the present, while the future on the other side gets his existence of predictions based on phenomena that exist in the present.

Despite these contradictions is Augustine's willing to accept the usual meaning of past, present and future and reason about how to be able to measure the time which passes the moment now. He indicates that it is possible to measure time with inspiration from astronomy to measure time with the movement of heavy bodies like the Sun, where the Sun's time in a day and a year can define time. When Augustine realizes the undefinable in time concept gives he proposed that it is the soul that would be made up in the eternal present. This issue of time and the experience of the

14

present moment are interesting in the context of how the brain's perception and consciousness sense our perception of "reality". Augustine's exposition on time (present, future and past) is subjective terms that can be linked to the human mental functions like perception (present), anticipation (future) and memory (past).

The nervous system

The brain's perception of time is shaped by a number of physiological properties of the human body. First a short simplified examination of the human nervous system's construction. It divides into the central nervous system (CNS, see fig. 1.1) consisting of the large brain (Cerebrum), Cerebellum and spinal cord, which is located in the spine. On the other hand, the peripheral nervous system (PNS) which is made up of all the nerve fibers that run in and out from the brain and spine cord which is associated with, among other things muscles and senses for sight, hearing, touch, smell and taste. The incoming signals from senses goes to the thalamus, which distributes the signals on to the different senses center of the cerebrum (see figure 1.3). Central nervous system takes the sensory signals from the peripheral nervous system and controls, among other things muscles and inner organ with motor output signals to the peripheral nervous system. The brain may through consciousness control e.g. skeletal muscle (somatic nervous system), while many activities in the body is controlled automatically, as for example heart and lungs via the autonomic nervous system.

The autonomic nervous system is in turn divided into the sympathetic nervous system, which acts in situations in which the body needs to be enabled in e.g. threats and the parasympathetic nervous system, which is activated in rest periods with the reconstruction and recovery of the body. Nervous systems are also linked to the endocrine system in the body that, among other things by the hypothalamus controls the different glands in the body via hormones in the blood system

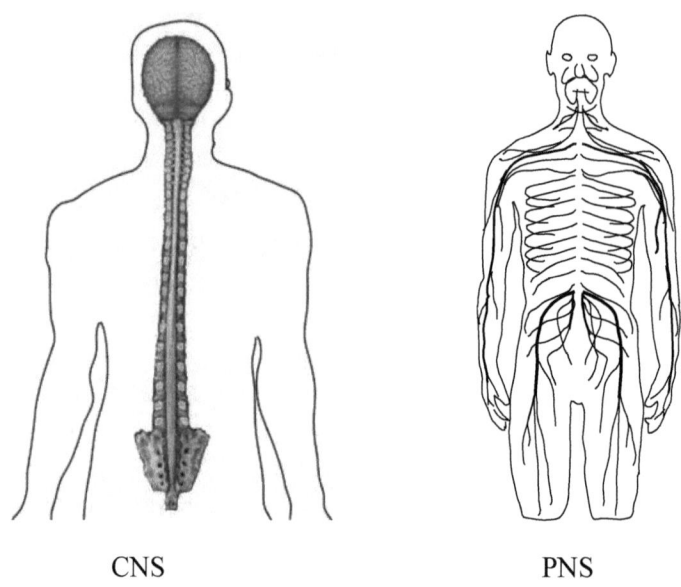

CNS   PNS

Fig. 1.1 Central and peripheral nerve system.

The brain weighs about 1.4 Kg and is made up of the cerebrum, brainstem and cerebellum, but despite the brain›s small size in the body it consumes ca 20% of the body›s total energy. The brain stem is the brain›s primitive part but takes care of many autonomous vital functions such as heart rate, breathing and even all incoming sensory information from the body›s senses (except the smell) that is distributed to various parts of the cerebrum where further processing continues. The cerebrum is divided into two hemispheres a left and right hemisphere where a deep longitudinal furrow separating them for and in its bottom is Corpus Callosum that connects the two cerebral hemispheres with an extensive networks. Each hemisphere are divided in frontal lobe, parietal lobe, temporal lobe and occipital lobe see figure 1.2.

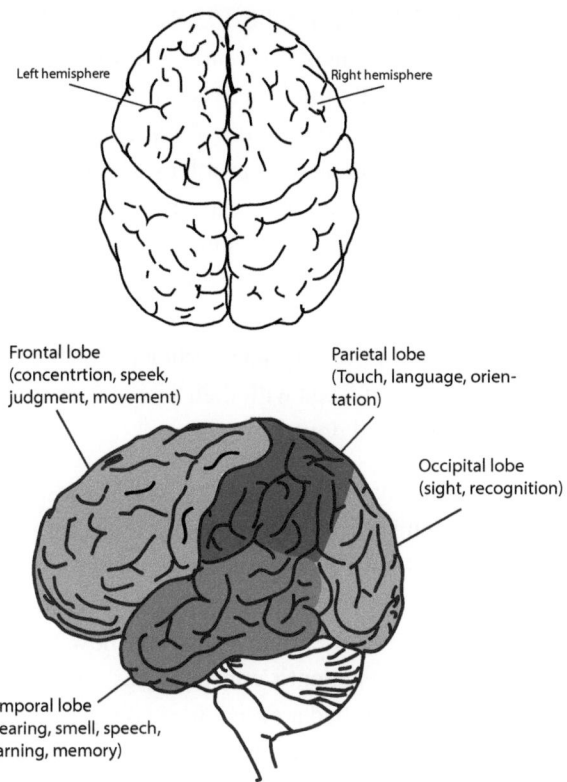

Left hemisphere

Right hemisphere

Frontal lobe
(concentrtion, speek,
judgment, movement)

Parietal lobe
(Touch, language, orien-
tation)

Occipital lobe
(sight, recognition)

Temporal lobe
(Hearing, smell, speech,
learning, memory)

Fig. 1.2 Brain anatomy, lobes

Each of the two cerebral hemispheres have different function than the left part is dominated in language, logic thinking, mathematics and detailed knowledge, while the right hemisphere instead has a better spatial perception, favoring creativity, spontaneity, musicality and gives a more holistic capability. Coordination of impressions in the two cerebral hemispheres is by the Corpus Callosum. The Corpus Callosum is crossed nerve pathways from the brain to the rest of the body where the left hemisphere controls the right half of the body (arms, legs , etc.) while the right hemisphere in the same way checks left body limbs. The majority of people who are right handed, have the left hemisphere as the dominant brain function and some believe that the mind in the first place is emanating from there.

When physician especially during the 1950's were performing operations on patients with severe epileptic seizures by cutting the nerve connections Corpus Callosum in the brain between the cerebral hemispheres they could remove or reduce the symptoms of patients ("split brain" procedures). As a side effect the patients got problem with the coordination of sensory input in the two brains hemispheres as in some cases could give the patient a sense of conflict between sense signals in the two hemispheres. The American neuro researcher Roger W Sperry (1913-1994) received the Nobel Prize in medicine in 1981 for his discoveries on the brains different features of left and right brain. Sperry had earlier in 1940 and 1950 s researched with animal testing on frogs with their vision nerves and partly on "split brain" surgery on cats and dogs.

Sperry got in the beginning of 1960's ability to make tests of the cognitive/mental ability of patients who undergone split brain surgery for curing severe epileptic seizures. One of the patients was a man who daily over a ten-year period suffered from severe seizures from injured in the earlier world war. Sperry designed test methods to identify how "split brain" the operation had an impact on the patient's consciousness and cognitive ability. Tests showed that the patient had a division of consciousness in the left and right hemisphere because that the information channel between the cerebral hemispheres had been cut.

In a first test series carried out early after surgery the patient was given a visual test where the subject had to fix his gaze on a midpoint on a monitor and then was shown various images on the left and right part of the screen for a short time. When the eye nerves partially crossover saw the left brain right and left eyes retinas right field of vision while the right hemisphere saw the right and left eyes retinas left field of vision. It was also in the test that the patient would pick up a similar object behind a screen with his right hand or left hand that had been displayed on the monitor (see Ref. 1.2, 1.3).

The result was that in the eye right field of vision could subject only perceived by the left hand and/or verbally, while in the eye left field of vision could object only be perceived with the right hand but not verbally. If both hands were left free to point out objects was chosen right hand for eye left field of view and the left hand in the eye right field of vision. Similar results had been at the tactile impact with a toothpick on right leg where the right arm could point out the contact point, while the left arm only had random designation. On the opposite side was the reverse to stimuli of the left leg could only single out with his left hand. The patient's location of tactile stimulation in the face, head and back of the head with both hands worked and could also be expressed verbally, which showed that these neural pathways follow the cranial nerve to this region. Sperry summarized the results as follows:

• Visual information was only available in the hemisphere that each eye right or left field of vision was linked to and only the same body's arm could point out the right items from the field of view

• Activities involving speech and writing worked only in the left hemisphere.

• Tactile influence followed the same pattern for left and right hemisphere that the visual information above, but tactile stimulation in the head region were intact and this could both sides point out stimuli sites and also provide verbal information.

• The result support earlier theory about the two hemispheres specialization there left hemisphere work better in talk, writing and logic while the right half is for spatial and artistic styles creativity.

• The Corpus Callosum in a normal brain Exchange information so that the necessary coordination of information between left and right hemisphere are available to consciousness.

It is a time delay of approximately 20 mS when stimuli are sent between the cerebral hemispheres through the Corpus Callosum.

The brain's higher mental functions are localized in the cerebral cortex which is the pleated layer which is surface on the cerebrum and is about 3-5 mm thick and contain very complex neural networks. Surface layer is grey and contains neurons links in different complex networks while matter in inside are white depending on the axon connection outputs from the neurons which is surrounded by myelin coat that has a white color. In addition to the approximately 100 billion neurons in the brain there are 10 times more different types of support cells that are referred to as glial cells. These cells support the second neurons with nutrition, immune system, form myelin coat, etc. The cerebral cortex contains a number of centers for, among other thing sense of touch, movement, language and higher mental functions including association areas for decision-making, logical reasoning and planning. This in order to process and combine all the information into an overall picture, which is why many believe that the human consciousness is shaped in the cerebral cortex.

The cerebellum (see fig. 1.3) sits at the bottom under the cerebrum in the back of the brain and is like the cerebrum divided into two hemispheres with pleated layers. The cerebellum will communicate with the cerebrum and spine-cord through the brainstem and the bridge (pons) with the help of numerous neural networks. You can see the cerebellum, among other things as a coordinator of the body's coordination movement, balance and control of the body posture. Fine motoric movements are monitored and rehearsed movement programs such as cycling, swimming or a somersault are stored in motion memories. When they have been practiced in is they left over long times as when you a time learned to ride a bike it last for the rest of the life. In a later chapter on body consciousness concerned cerebellar function in pursuit of budo-sports.

Communication via spinal cord contains information from receptors in muscles, joints and tendons on their mutual positions of control of movement and posture. From the brainstem are signals from balance cores and motor skills. By nuclei in pons are signaling from the brain-cortex sensory and motor cortex received. Research has also indicated that movement programs probably created in an "internal model" of trained operating projects in the cerebellum. Incoming perception from the body's sensors are compared with the internal model's status to be able to continuously correct the deviation. If reported deviations are too large for normal correction is called movement center in the cerebral cortex for intervention. Normally releases the cerebellum cerebrum from routine work with micro-management by body motions' as in for example normal driving by a skilled driver offloads much brain work. Later time research showing that in addition to regulation of motor body movements, processes in our thinking and our emotions are managed in the cerebellum that dealing with numbers, speaking and writing on an ongoing basis with the fluency of movements.

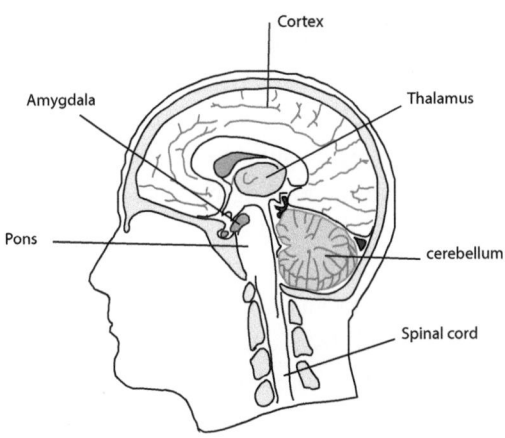

Fig. 1.3 The brains anatomy

The nerve cell

A neuron cell which is the basis of the brain and nervous system have in detail a very complex composition, which is outside this book detail level, but it provides a rough description of the most important parts of a neurons. In figure 1.4 shows a simplified picture of the neuron structure. Like all cells in the body is deep down a nucleus which contain the genetic code for the cell's biology. The surfaces of the cell are the membrane that forms the boundary for the area. Some important protrusions from the cell membrane is on one hand, they often many short spiky protrusions called dendrites which is the port for the signals from the environment and secondly the only long protrusion called axon, which is the cell's output as connected to the next neuron.

Inside the neuron is signaling by nerve impulses through electricity and between a cell axon and the next cells dendrite is a structural unit which is called the synapse and which give signal through the release of chemical neurotransmitters. These signal substances (neurotransmitters) such as acetylcholine is a signal substance usually seen in central nerve system synapses. The signal path is: electrical-chemical-electrical...;. The electrical signal is generated chemically in the neuron cell and gives a voltage of around -70 mV between in and outside of the cell membrane in the rest. Activation of a nerve cell by a dendrite is made through a chemical reaction the exchange of sodium ions Na + and potassium ions K + in the cell through ports in cell membrane whereby voltage is approximately + 30 mV on the inside (see figure 1.5). After that there are made a reset to the cell's rest voltage -70 mV, through a new gear ratio of sodium ions and potassium ions through the gates in the cell membrane.

As figure 1.5 shows a voltage pulse that propagates through axon to next nerve cells synapse and releases signal and this voltage pulse called the action potential. The receiving nerve cell receptors at the synapse that is susceptible to the current signal substance (neurotransmitter) and if the cell is stimulated with sufficient amount of signal substance occurs also in this cell an action potential which via its axon is sent to the next nerve cell. The impulse can then go through many nerve cells before it e.g. provides a response in a muscle. There are also neurotransmitters which instead can inhibit a cell in to bring a nerve impulse in nerve chain.

The cell can therefore only deal with one nerve impulse at time before a new one can be generated, which means that if a nerve fiber is activated during a certain period of time it sent pulsing with nerve signals that the interval between pulses determines the intensity of such as a muscle activation. An increased frequency of pulses gives greater activity in the muscle cell, see fig. 1.6. When the signal of stimuli by the nerve fiber is a combination of electrical signals and chemical transfer between neurons in a nerve chain will signals to be delayed various long upon arrival to the brain's sensing center. This is depending by how long the signal path a nerve fiber has for example from a toe or from the nose.

Back in the 1840's, the German scientist Hermann Holmberg measurements on a frog leg for measuring the nerve signal propagation speed and came up to about 30 m/s in a frog. When it comes to a person's nerve the out signal delay from the nerve cell's axon depends on wing of diameter on the axon and if it have a surrounding body cote called myelin. One can roughly divide the nerve fibers in three categories:

• A-fiber: Fast, up to 150 m/s, (rough, myelin) is included in e.g. motor neurons.

• B-fiber: Half speed, about 15 m/s, (medium pile, easy myelin) included in e.g. sensor from the skin.

• C-fiber: Slow, about 1 m/s, (thin, not myelin) according to previous.
Generally, we say that the rough of quick nerve fibers connecting the nerve pathways from for example feet and legs (for example. sciatic nerve) which provides faster transmission on the relatively long pathway to the brain.

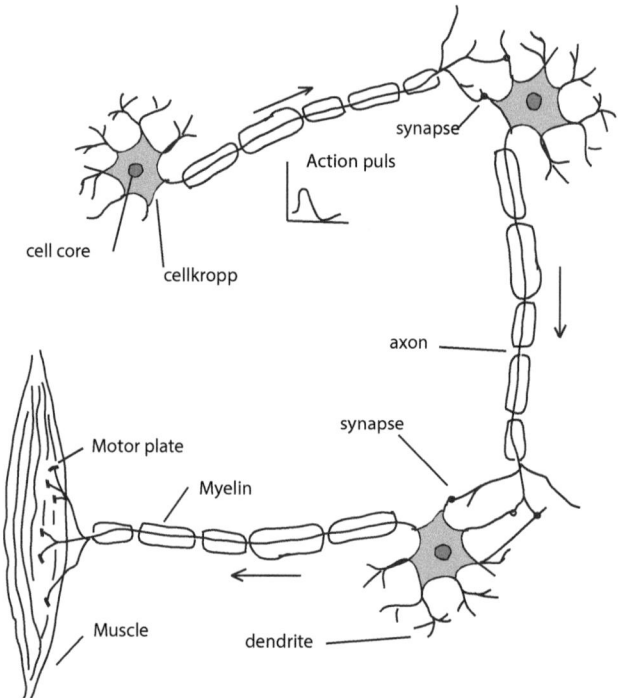

Fig. 1.4 Nerve cell anatomy and function

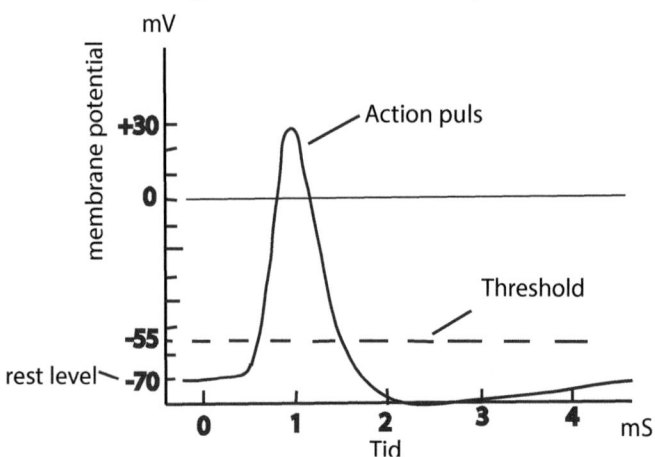

Fig. 1.5 Neuron action potential.

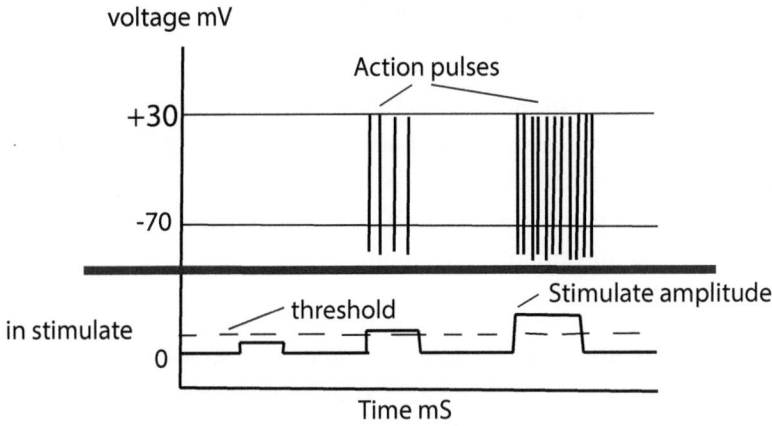

Fig. 1.6 Propagation of nerve signals

The image of a neuron in figure 1.4 is just a general basic picture of motor neuron, while it in the body is a number of different types of nerve cells which are structurally and functionally different. When it comes to so-called afferenta nerve fibers, which results in nerve impulses to the brain by spinal cord, there are a number of different types this result in nerve impulses for control of the body's external environment, the body's internal environment, body movement and body posture. Below is reported some important types of these nerve cells.

• Mechanoreceptors: React on squeeze, vibration or strain, during sound, body position, blood pressure or touch.

• Heatreceptors: react to temperature changes in the skin and the hypothalamus. Some register cooling other heat.

• Chemoreceptors: react to change in the chemical environment including the blood's content of oxygen and carbon dioxide, while others respond to odors or flavors

• Photo receptors: reacting to the incident visible light with cones and rods in the fundus (electromagnetic waves).

• Nociceptor: Pain receptors, reacts on tissue damage in the skin, articular capsule, periosteum or blood vessels.

The skin's nerve pathways for tactile areas (dermatomes) led by spine cord to special areas in the large cerebral cortex (somatosensory cortex). Where can you locate areas for each nerve connections that form a map of the body's different skin area. Level of details depends on e.g. that a finger have many neural pathways for sensitive motor skills, while other areas of skin give coarser information (see figure 1.7).

Heat receptors works in increasing range of 30 – 50 degrees and report pain at temperatures above about 45degrees centigrade. Cold receptors works in the fall range 10 - 45 degrees and is reporting pain at temperature below about 15 degrees centigrade. Nociceptor providing pain perception when damage and has two types of nerve fibers , on the one hand A-delta fibers that provide a sharp cutting located pain with relative high speed (5 - 25 m/s) and C fibers, which gives a more dull non located pain in lower speed (0.1 – 2 m/s).

It is a number of built-in protective reflexes in the nervous system for example nee jerk which is triggered by a kind of patella reflexes under the kneecap and tested often in the context of the medical examination. Similarly triggered rapid reflexes of nociceptors in the sole of the foot throw the leg away from the pain if you step on a nail or on a hot land surface. These reflexes is not through the brain's motor skills but switched over directly in spine cord to avoid damage, then the detour by the nerve signals to the brain and consciousness would take too long.

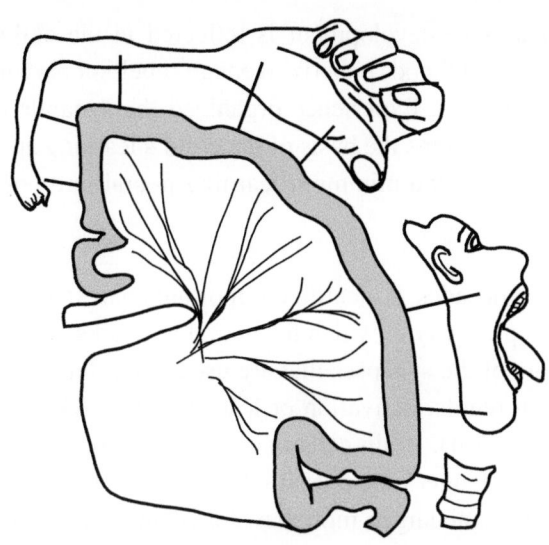

Fig. 1.7 Homunculus, chart nerve areas in somatosensoty cortex.

Brain plasticity

The developments of the brains of vertebrates are made out of three embryonic blisters. In humans these three blisters developed to the cerebrum, brainstem, and pons/cerebellum/spinal cord. Due to the brain's complexity is man's childhood and youth development very long compare brought with the rest of the animal world. We are born with approximately 100 billion neurons in the brain, but the neural network between neurons must be built up through physical exercise and cognitive learning for many years. Already the motor learning for a child from that first just moving arms and legs for that then crawl before they practiced up balance and can walk requires years of practice.

These regions for movements and sensory analysis are myelinated first and then for up to twenty-five years of age the last parts of the fraotal lob in the brain, which controls the higher function of the brain, is myelinated.

This brain's successive development is reflected in the child's different ages with the first childhood, puberty, teenage rebellion and maturity first in twenty-five years old. Experience organized the synaptic connections between neurons and forms the basis of the child's learning and adaptation to environment, where the minimum learning neural unit consists of the synapse.

During the last decades, it identified important context about what is referred to as brain plasticity in which the neural networks are being worked through the purge of the synapses that are used at least and how new synapses grow out at regular activation or learning of new knowledge, "Use it or lose it ", (Ref. 1.4). Brain cells that do not receive any contact with another cells over a longer time dies at idle in the brain. Active training allows the nerves become larger, more developed and better connected with each other. This plasticity in the brain is largest in the beginning of life when the immature brain organizes it selves. But even in the case of a brain injury, in which new nerve connections can compensate for lost functions and also in adult age when new things are learned, there are built connections with new synapses.

Example of brain plasticity is what happens if one for example in the event of an accident loses a hand. A hand has great representation in the brain's somatosensory cortex and when hand's projection will be silenced this area of free and unused. The brain accepts not this quiet area but within a short time grows neuronal connections from surrounding areas for the face and the other arm into in this hand's previous area (see figure 1.7). In some cases, the person experiencing phantom pain from the loss of his hand. For example, this may give a touch of the face the same feeling like sensory experiences from the previous hand. Phantom pains can sometimes be intolerable and depends on the size of the intervention of new nerve connections become in the hands previous area. One way to reduce phantom pain is that the patient is exercising his healthy hand next to a parallel mirror. The patient sees a picture in the mirror as if the amputated hand exists left and can be moved. Repeated training with this method can restore the body map in neocortex and reduce phantom pains.

At research using fMRI which tested the brain regions that are activated during exercise for faster motor reaction time, the researcher had been able to measuring that the corresponding brain regions are active during the following night's REM sleep. This indicates that it builds up new connections through synapses in the corresponding network during the recovery period. Research (Ref. 1.5) at The Sahlgrenska Academy in Goteborg has demonstrated that it is connection between young people who have been training their physical fitness and thus rated better on IQ tests. The survey was made on the 1.2 million male conscripts' born1950 to 1976, which in conjunction with patterning (age 18) underwent physical and cognitive IQ tester. It was found in a long term study a clear connection between higher academic training and positions in working life for those who had better physical fitness at patterning. An effect is believed to be that a good heart/lung capacity can provide good conditions for the brain's basic supply.

In this context, it may be of interest to highlight how complex our neural networks is to be able to keep the human body upright in the balance, to be able to walk and run. By trying to balance a regular pencil on a finger realize to how complex it is for a long man to balance the body not to fall to ground in the Earth's gravity field. This is efferenta motor neuron for the regulation and distribution of muscle tension involved together with afferenta sensor neurons in order to get feedback from balance organ in the inner ear. In this loop is also muscle receptors involved witch gives feedback of muscle position, stretched and change of speed. When these nerve pathways must be coordinated in order to get stability, one can see the motor system as a control system which by feedback can be made stable but also requires that these neural pathways are fast (80-120 m/s), why they are myelinated.

Because past activities with digital signal processing in flying radar system, have I experience of the complexity in that get a feedback-system to be stable. An aircraft may as well as the human body move itself in three dimensions and to control a radar antenna to lock on to a target, we must on the one hand, measure the input from tracking and both provide control commands to the antenna in millisecond place and in addition, you will need reinforcement in the regulation must be selected with attention to amplification for the system to avoid oscillations or got too much time delay.

In the human body are handled this control by the brain's motor cortex, somatosensory cortex, cerebellum, brain stem and via spine cord nerve pathways to each muscle group in the limbs (see fig. 1.9). For a child it takes a long time to train up the balance to be able to stand upright. When we walk or run will affect the body's Center of gravity to end up outside of the balance point, which must be compensated by taking steps forward or backward, which entails a complex control of the motor system. All this execution is handled normally unconsciously, but can be done deliberately by the intervention via somatic nervous system. In figure 1.8 shows a strongly simplified diagram of the structures that are involved in the body's balance control. The vestibular system in the ears provides information about the body's position and movement. Eye muscles are controlled in order to stabilize the field of view by movement. Proprioceptors in calf muscles give information about the body's position and movement. The cerebellum acts as a coordinating function for the fine motor movements. When you are standing still is a major signaling to and from the calf muscles which rhythmically compensates muscle tension in your calf muscles to stabilize the balance.

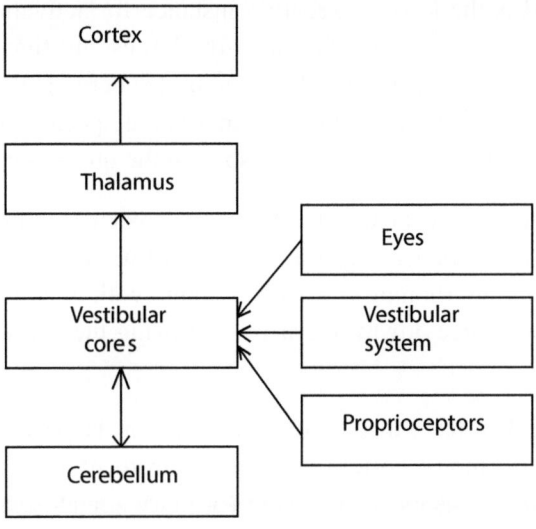

Fig. 1.8 Balance system in the brain

The complex control system of the body by walking and running requires on-making unconscious activities in the motor system. In figure 1.9 shows in simplified block diagram of the structures involved in the motor system's rules system.

One can divide the movement system in three hierarchical levels according to the figure.

• Spine cord is the lowest execution instance for activation and feed-back attached to muscles for reflexes, eurhythmics and time. Then it requires fast signal transfer is carried out the motor nerve pathways of type A-Alpha motor neuron with about 100 m/s range speed. Feedback from muscle proprioceptors are carried out also with the quick nerve paths.

• The next level is located in the brain stem where a number of cores assigned to vision, balance organ and postural muscle control from proprioceptors (walking, running) is involved along with fine tuning from the cerebellum. The coarse downward arrows showing the nerves for muscle control.

• The cerebral cortex which contains centers for the basic muscle management (primary motor cortex) and centers from proprioceptors in the muscles and other sensors such as skin (primary somatosensory cortex). These two centers are located in the middle of the brain tight with limbs represented order with feet at the top and head at the bottom (see figure 1.10). For planning and control of movements are several association areas in the cortex: for planning of movement and mirroring (premotor cortex), willed sequences (additional own motor cortex), will control (prefrontal cortex), and integration of, among other things spatial sensations (parietal cortex).

As the block diagram shows, this control system is extremely complicated and requires a very large computing capacity at about 3 billion of nerve pulses/second. It have recently in the United States managed to take up a robot skeleton (ReWalk) that can be worn by a paralyzed person and give the person the opportunity to take shorter walks. Still, this robot skeleton has great difficulty in managing the balance at the time of stairs. This review of the body's operating system is not profound but wants to give a certain understanding of the complexities of the body's movement as background for future description of the human experience of time courses among others, depending on the delays found in nerve communication.

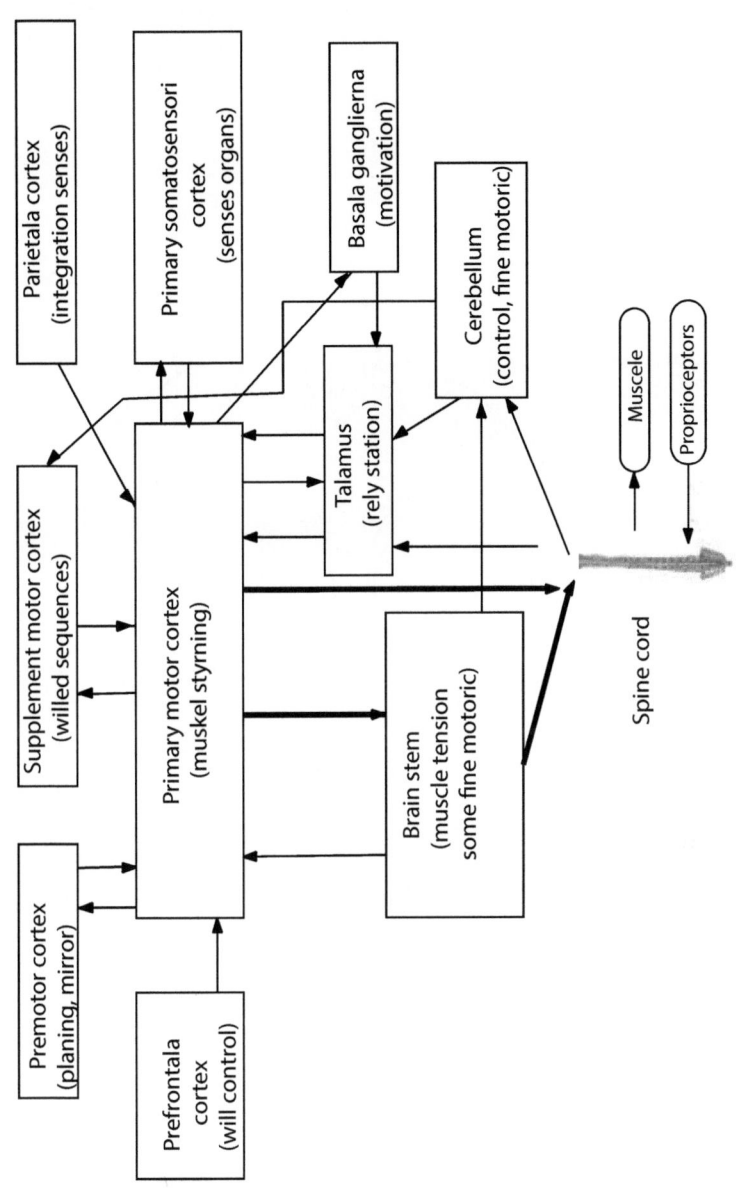

Fig. 1.9 Control of the motoric system.

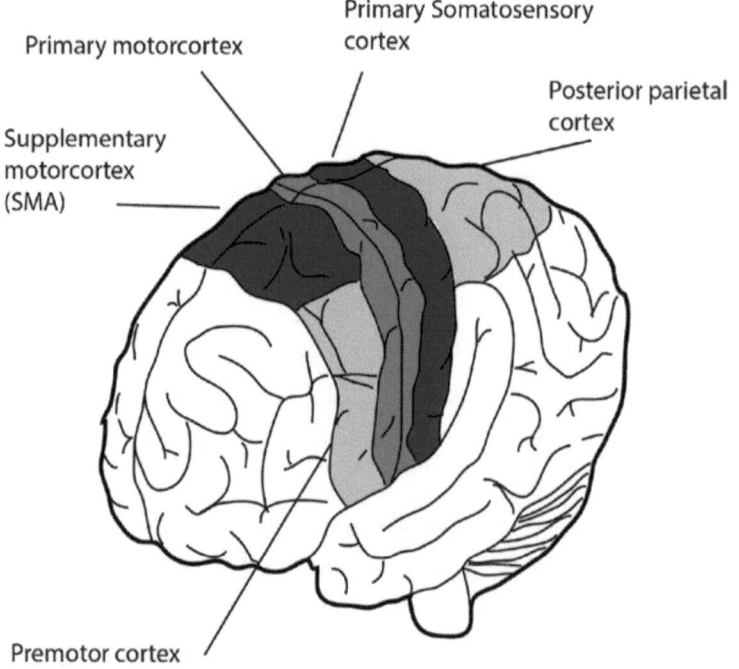

Fig. 1.10 Anatomy of motoric control.

The brains sense of time

With starting point in Augustine's description of the present time as the transition between history and future, we have to think about how we as human experiencing "the real moment now", with the delays our neural pathways have. At the end of 1800 and the beginning of the 20th century interested scientists to measure up the nerve path speeds and came up to the need for at least 10 to 20 milliseconds for sensor signals to reach the brain. The psychiatrist Hans Berger discovered 1929 (Ref. 1.6) that you could measure the electrical phenomena of the brain with electrodes attached to the scalp which was the prototype for today's electroencephalography, EEG. This resulted in a large progress to be able to measure activity in the brain's neurons (see further in chapter about biofeedback). The method is relatively rough then the required tasks in a greater number of nerve cells to provide a measurable result on the outside of the skull. One way to isolate a particular activity can be to implement many similar such operating torque and make an integration of measures to streamline the results of a specific desired activity.

Two scientists Hans Kronhuber and Lyder Deecke interested themselves in order to measure the state of the brain at various activities and used the EEG equipment in the experiment (1964) for measuring brain waves when the subject performed a spontaneous movement with his hand or foot (see ref. 1.7). A large number of measurements were made with 12 healthy subjects with a 100 number measurements for each person. At analysis of EEG data discovered researchers a special slow growing negative pulse of the order of 10 - 15 Microvolt (in the supplementary motor cortex area, SMA) prior to movement by e.g. bending of a finger. In figure 1.11 shows a basic picture of that pulse that came to be called readiness potential. What surprised the researchers was that this pulse slowly built up from about 1 second before the movement was carried out despite the fact that the subject himself decided as the movement would be carried out. This unconscious activity before the consciousness of movement starting led in a discussion if we as humans have a conscious free will or is controlled by unconscious processes in the brain.

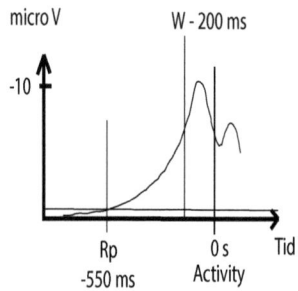

Fig. 1.11 Rp= readiness potential, W= conscioues decision.

A few epoch-making progress in brain research when it comes to how human consciousness sorts out the most important nerve signals from the huge influx of 11 M bit/s signals, which comes from our five senses in addition to all internal nerve signals were taken by researcher Benjamin Libet (1916-2007) a professor of neurophysiology at the University of California. The most remarkable discovery was that human consciousness is delayed approximately 0.5 seconds in relation to a way in for example the senses from skin of a hand. This shows how complex the human experience of to be in the present moment are, which already Augustine said. This is the basis of the so called "binding problem" which sets the question how consciousness can join all events in the brain's nervous system which is localized in different parts of the cerebral cortex with the perceived time factor.

Already in the 1930's mapped surgeon Wilder Penfield how the body's different parts were attached to the somatosensory cortex and motor cortex in the context of the patients underwent surgery for epileptic seizures. Benjamin Libet who was close friend of neurosurgeon Bertram Feinstein at Mount Zion hospital in San Francisco got the opportunity with the patient's permission to examine patients who underwent Stereotactic brain surgery during the 1960 's where the brain was accessible through that hole was taken up in the skull. Through the discovery of readiness potential at the motor movement Libet was interested of the relationship between the electrical activities that proceeded in SMA before it made the action became aware.

Then the cortex itself does not have any nerves for sensation or pain could Libet with electrodes provide electrical pulses to the various structures in somatosensory cortex which of the patient was conscious as different tingling or sensations in the corresponding body part as for example in a hand (see ref. 1.8). Libet noted that in order to a patient would be a aware for example of a stitch in a hand have the electrical pulse train last during at least 0.5 seconds otherwise experienced the person no stimulation (each individual pulse about 1 ms).

Libet published more research findings in 1967 (see Ref. 1.9) where via electrodes directly into the cortex could measure weak EEG signals when you for example stimulated skin on one hand. The results showed that much weak stimulation of the skin as the patient did not become aware of could give a nerve pulse in cerebral cortex which could be measured in EEG registration and these electrical impulses known as "evoked potentials" (see fig. 1.12). Although Libet informed the patient of the stimulation the patient felt no conscious stimulation although evoked potential could be measured. In his report in Science 1967 noted Libet that this relationship would be a physiological explanation for the sensation "subliminal perception".

Libet noted two different phenomena from their experiments and to a change in the EEG (evoked potential) can occur without reaching consciousness and an electrical stimulation in cerebral cortex require half-second duration for to reach consciousness. Libet asked on the issue if it consciously experiencing the half second stimulation when it occurs or after the half seconds passed. In a report in the Brain, 1979 (see ref. 1.10) described Libet an experiment for that determines when the patient experiences conscious stimulation. Libet put up the attempt as he stimulated a stitch in one hand directly into the cerebral cortex, while stimulating the skin on the other hand. The patient would respond with the hand that he was aware of only the left, right, or both at the same time. Libet made a number of attempts to change the sequence and time between stimulation of the two areas.

The result of the experiments surprised then the expectation that if stimulation via the cortex was going on would this consciously experienced after 0.5 s while a later started stimulation of the skin should be experienced later. Instead, the experiment showed that skin stimulation was perceived before the cortex stimulation even after up to 0.4 s delay relatively brain barks-simulation. Libets's conclusion was that the mind is projected back in time and is perceived as to be experienced in connection with its evoked potential, but with a direct stimulation of the cerebral cortex that is an unnatural stimulation does not produce any reversal in the subjective experience of time. You could call such a mechanism to be a correction for the built in delay in the brain's consciousness.

Libet performed additional experiments to ensure his theory by providing stimulation by nerves in the thalamus and there found same result that it took 0.5 s before stimulation was conscious but that even in this case may an evoked potential of cerebral cortex as the patient's consciousness is related in time to the evoked potential.

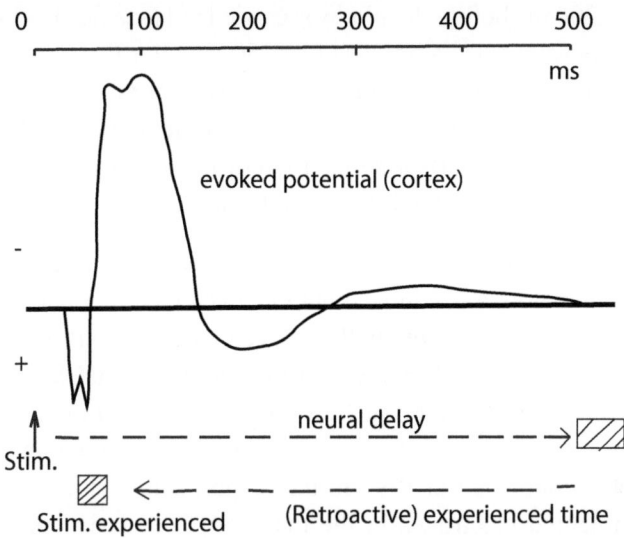

| 0 | 100 | 200 | 300 | 400 | 500 |

ms

evoked potential (cortex)

neural delay

Stim.

Stim. experienced   (Retroactive) experienced time

Fig. 1.12 Evoked potential, återmatning av upplevd tid.

Libet did also experiment with starting point in the previously mentioned readiness potential which can be measured up with the EEG in the cerebral cortex by execution of body movements. The starting point was to try to clarify any action when you deliberately perform a movement. When will readiness's potential occurs, when is the decision taken and when performed the action? Attempts were made in 1979 with five healthy volunteers as instructed to wait to start bending a finger until he himself got the desire to do it (see Ref. 1. 11). EMG signals from the finger showed when the action was done, EEG signals from cortex council of the SMA was measured in order to see readiness potential and a special oscilloscope with a bright dot that rotated around the periphery with speed 2.56 seconds per lap that volunteers would note to mark time when he took his decision to act. A scale with resolution 60 lines was around the edge and each line corresponded to about 43 milliseconds.

The results showed that readiness potential entering 550 milliseconds (ms) before handling and observation of oscilloscopes clock at decision time was 200 ms before the plot was carried out (see fig. 1. 11). This means that the conscious decision feels like 350 ms after that readiness potential has started. Therefore an unconscious activity starts 350 ms before you experience to take the decision on the action! Libet finds that the brain apparently unknowingly starts a preparation of the action until we consciously perceived to have taken a decision on the action.

Libet results partly on the delay of 0.5 s and the unconscious activity in the brain before e.g. a movement of a hand has started an intense debate about if the man has a free will or governed by unconscious processes in the brain. Libet himself has stated that the prefrontal lobes in the brain have a veto power against such as a plot by the 200 ms that precedes an action is carried out and thus can prevent a possible unconscious bad action. Libet conducted in 1991 further experiments with patients endowed with implanted electrodes in the thalamus to electric impetus moderate severe chronic pain perception. By stimulating these electrodes in the thalamus with pulsing shorter or longer than the half second that it takes for to be aware if a stimulation could Libet verify their previous results that it required a minimum of 0.5 s duration of stimulation before it becomes conscious (Ref. 1.12). In addition, the patient was able to "guess right" to stimulation going on if the stimulation was between 0.25-0, 5 although no conscious stimulation felt. This suggests that we can perceive "subliminal perception" for shorter stimuli than 0.5 s then it performs an evoked potential in the brain.

Libet experiments with the mechanisms when making a spontaneous motion with his finger, has recently been repeated 2011 where new methods with the help of fMRI and especially high magnetic fields (7 tesla) used which can give a more detailed magnetic x-ray picture of activity in the cerebral cortex. Professor John-Dylan Haynes at the Max Planck institute for human cognitive and brain sciences in Leipzig has performed experiments with 12 subjects who would choose between to press down a mouse button either to the right or the left index finger when he himself requested (see ref. 1.16). For that time relate when the person became aware of the decision appeared a random sequence of letters on a screen at the rate of 2 Hz, so, 500 ms, where the person was asked to relate the letter that appeared when the decision was deliberate. It was stressed that the subject would be relaxed and more randomly chooses when button pressure would take place. At in difference from Libet chose Haynes that specifically examines parts of the prefrontal cortex which is considered to represent the upper hierarchical level in cerebral cortex. In this area, see among others. Information from somatosensory cortex for control of conscious movements (sympathetic nervous system), will control, business intelligence, planning and motivation. In comparison with Libet try where EEG registration used for measurement of readiness potential in SMA 550 milliseconds before activity, is expected activity in the prefrontal cortex unconscious much earlier in the chain. The results showed that the increased activity in the prefrontal cortex started in 7 seconds before the task's execution, i.e. long before the subject became aware that a decision has been taken. Through refined analysis of blood flow to the prefrontal cortex could even to 100 % determine what key the subject would press on. Thus confirms this study Libet previous results to this type of decision is taken by unconsciousness processes in the brain and that consciousness will come later, which poses the question of man's free will to a head.

Despite the built-in delay of approx. 0.5 S of consciousness we can often be trained through automatic movements of about 0.2-0.3 S react time. As skilled drivers notice sometimes that intuitively makes a quick deceleration without knowingly have taken such a decision, probably depending on that we subliminally detected an incoming obstacles far out in the peripheral field of view and thereby avoided a collision. In the sports context e.g., in tennis, the ball's speed so high that a player must act fairly instinct to be able to return a hard battles serve. Another aspect that affects us as people in the experience of the present day, is our inability to distinguish the stimuli coming from, among other things our sight, hearing and sense of touch due to the neural lag. When it comes to sights requires process to shape a conscious visual order of 0.1 second. If the laboratory tests showing flashing lights can motion be an illusion by operating at the appropriate frequency and the distance between the lamps. This is used for example in wandering inscriptions where matrix of lamps shapes text that seems to glide across the screen.

The same phenomenon is behind that we can perceive motion in cinema films that appear with 24 frames per second with a short black space or television -images with image frequency 50 Hz. One can compare to the early silent films that had a slow display with about 12 frames per second when the movements looked very twitchy and quick out. Our vision of "reality" contains simulations where for example the blind spot in the eye (where the optic nerve passes out) simulated away in the conscious field of view. It is also a lot of examples of images where the brain identifies various sensations of objects and sometimes registering the same picture on several different ways. Similar delays are also in other sensory sensations such as hearing and sense of touch.

Consciousness

There is an intense debate about how our consciousness arises, but still only a number of theories which not scientifically has been able to be verified. Consciousness is in deep sleep, when you get put to sleep during an operation, or are in a coma disconnected and return on waking. Researcher Giulio Tononi that research on sleep and consciousness at the University of Wisconsin-Madison have in experiments with TMS (Transcranial Magnetic Stimulation) done experiments with subjects whose brains have been examined with EEG first in the awake state. Then a person induced by TMS a directed magnetic field to a central part of the cerebral cortex, there are increased blood-flow only in the target area and immediately thereafter propagated it to other centers in the cortex. When the subject is exposed for the same stimulus with TMS in deep sleep so get one again an increased blood flow to target area, but propagation to other areas in the cortex may not appear. This could indicate that the neural networks in the brain cortex are involved in generation of consciousness. But to go into the deeper details, there are two schools on how a consciousness arises where the one advocating a dualistic interpretation of consciousness while the other advocates that consciousness is in the physical structure neural network.

Professor David Chalmers of the University of California has in an article in 1995 descibed the awareness problem by to specify the problem that on the one hand, the simple problem and, on the other hand, the difficult problem (see ref. 1.13). Chalmers said that the simple problem involves a number of observable cognitive properties: the ability to recognize, categorize and respond to external stimuli, integration of information in the cognitive system, interpret of mental states, the possibility of focusing of attention, control of behavior and the difference between wakefulness and sleep. The difficult problem is our internal experiences of "qualia" as when we have visual or audio experiences where the feeling of the color deep blue or the tone (C) introduces a subjective quality that is unique to each individual. Chalmers ask why causes the cognitive processes opportunities for a private inner life and not just a direct reaction to incoming stimuli automatically or as a "zombie". He asks questions about the subjective experiences "in an inner life" would only be functions of the neural network or if you need new theories with non-physical background. Chalmers suggests that it must be undiscovered new fundamental laws corresponding to the mass and time that could explain the inner experiences of the knowledge. Professor of philosophy Daniel Dennett at Tufts University (United States) is one of the philosophers who believe that Chalmers difficult problem comes from an invalid thought experiment and believe that the difficult problem can be reduced to the behavior and judgement. In contrast to Chalmers, Dennett believes that the mind is not a fundamental property of the universe, but is likely to be explained by natural phenomena in brain networks. Dennett also believe that the simple and difficult problem has to be solved jointly because they constitute a coherent par.

In this issue of consciousness had researcher Benjamin Libet own theory where he in an article suggested the presence of a consciousness field (consciousness mental field, CMF) without physical neural pathways which were could be an explanation as to the subjective experience of consciousness that we as human are experiencing (see Ref. 1.14). Libet proposed an experiment in which the operative cut of the neural connections (axons) to an isolated area of the brain with intact nutrition could measure if no CMF activity could take place between this area and the associated brain area. Libet argued that if such a field would exist, is it not a sign of a dualistic theory because the field would require a living brain to exist.

Other researchers e.g. professor Wolf Singer at the Max-Planck-Institute for Brain Research in Frankfurt believe that consciousness is created in the physical structure of neocortical neural network. Singer has made fundamental discoveries in experiments on the sense of sight of, among other thing cats and monkeys which would be able to explain the so called "binding problem ". Binding problem raises the question of how consciousness arises from all the different regions of the cerebral cortex that in parallel on their own processes were processing perception, which is compiled to a person's overall experience of consciousness. Singer has in an article "Binding by synchrony" described discoveries in connection with the research on the sense of sight in cats with the help of implanted multiple electrodes in the cat visual cortex (see ref.1.15). At experiment with moving black and white squares in the field of view of the cats discovered synchronous oscillations between spatial different brain regions with frequency 40 Hz (gamma waves) that was different from the normal activity for seeing. The researchers believed that this oscillation and synchronize had its background in neurons communication via networks. This led to the hypothesis that the neural networks used synchronize in millisecond tact for the activities of groups of neurons which thus can dynamically transmit coded information by the neural network. As we have seen in the past have neurons a special timeline for the generation of action potential (see figure 1.5), where the triggering of a pulse action via dendrites are sensitive in the initial phase, while it prevented in the downward phase. This can lead that incoming pulses which is synchronous with the neuron action potential can give increased pulsing when incoming signals have the right phase in millisecond tact. According to Singer has more research in several laboratory with multiple methods of measurement in cerebral cortex strengthened the hypothesis that a variety of cognitive functions such as: grouping of perception, focusing of attention, treatment of impressions in short term memory, integration of sensory perception, formation of associative memories and sensory coordination can have a close relationship with synchronous oscillating signals in frequency area of the Beta and Gamma in the neural network (approximately 13 Hz, 40 Hz).

There are more theories on how binding problem works and about how consciousness arise, but today there is no common accepted scientific explanation for the phenomenon of consciousness. Some see binding problem from two aspects, as the problem how the brain can pick up individual items from the complex patterns from, for example view the input to distinguish a blue square and a yellow circle, but not confuse their color. On the other hand, the combinatorial problem to coordinate how an object and its background can be interpreted with emotional experiences and be combined into a common experience (external view).

Consciousness is of course also a system with the ability to consider and eamine his own mirror image. This is an indication of a hierarchy of consciousness where higher functions can examine the underlying functionality and that for example in later chapter on hypnosis shows themselves selectively to close of the higher perception of signals from our minds to consciousness. Hopefully, the ongoing research and the mapping of the brain's neurological network that was mentioned in the beginning of the chapter can contribute to the understanding of the mechanisms and origins.

At the end of this chapter presents two important discoveries on the neural network. In the rest, researcher are interested to measure the spontaneous fluctuations in the brain's cortex, which is caused by streams of consciousness such as daydreams, forward planning and thoughts of past events (episodic memory). Already in 1974, complained of the Swedish scientist professor David Ingvar that was a high activity in the brain's prefrontal lobe even in the rest. At that time he used xenon 133 inhalation techniques for measurement of regional blood flow in the brain (rCBF). Ingvar argued that a rise in activity in the rest occurred in specific regions of the brain, where especially the prefrontal lobes were included.

These early findings were confirmed by the researcher Marcus Raichle, professor of Neurology at the Washington University in St. Louis. Raichle coined the term "default network" in a research report published in Nature reviews Neuroscience 2001 (ref. 1.17). This report describes Raichle for his research on brain metabolism at rest and mental strain. The results showed that the brain's energy consumption by passivity and activity differ only 5 %. FMRI measurements showed that the continued high activity in the brain even during rest especially between the frontal lobe and the parietal lobe. These networks have then been explored more in detail and referred to "Default network". The research showed that when an external stimulus from environment was caught or problem-solving going on in brain activity to was shifted in different centers. Activity in the default network decreased and ruled on to the new task area. Through to take difference in blood flow between the fMRI images from dormant condition and for example during visual fixation showed the result of increased activity in the visual cortex. In the same way could activity when reading words point out increased activity in brain areas of language. In later years, they have been able to see that this default network is affected by a number of neurological disorders such as schizophrenia, autism and Alzheimer's. At schizophrenia is an overload of activity in the parietal lobe that can give hallucinations or paranoia. At autism has a lower activity in the default network than among healthy people. At Alzheimer's disease can be also noted that the default network is damaged by plaque which affect synapses.

In the context of the research project "the human connectome project" has researcher discovered some central areas in the cortex which have especially powerful neural network between themselves. In this research there are three different approaches to the neural network. Basic research on the anatomy of the networks is done using the DTI (Diffusion tensor imaging) where you document networks extent via water molecules diffusion along neuronal axons. When it comes to networks functional connections used methods with EEG, MEG and fMRI for localization of cortex functional centers. The third method analyzes the effectiveness of the link nerve cells in between. Analysis of the brain's total network can be divided into several hierarchical levels as: individual neurons, local clusters of neurons and clusters of neurons in anatomically distinct brain areas. Through comparisons between structural and functional studies can for example fMRI measurements find correlations between the networks and the current brain function. When it comes to networks effectiveness of clutches need the dynamics of the temporal signals views through the appropriate time measurements.

The two scientists Olaf Sporns and Martijn van den Heuvel published 2011 an article in the Journal of Neuroscience about new research on brain network (see ref. 1.18). In a study of 21 subjects were made DTI measurements for 30 minutes where the person was in dormant state. The researcher reviewed 82 different centers in the brains and mapped their neural network. The two scientists located 12 different centers that had twice the nerve connections in their networks than the other centers. In addition, these centers unusually have many nerve connections in networks with each other. In addition these centers are primarily involved in higher cognitive functions in the brain. The researchers called these 12 centers for "rich club" and believe that these networks can be the source of man's consciousness and the emergence of "I"-feeling. The 12 centers are located in 6 centers in each hemisphere (see fig. 1.13). The Centre with the most connections are area precuneus, which is an area in the back of the brain. This area is not detailed mapped but are assumed to have an integrative function for information from many centers in the brain. The second area is the superior frontal cortex which is involved in planning and control attention. Third area is superior parietal cortex as in-hold visual information about the visual object's position. The fourth area is the hippocampus, which manages the storage and access of memories. The fifth area is the thalamus which, among other things is involved in Visual information. Finally, the sixth area is putamen as, among other things coordinates the motions. The researchers believe that this "rich club" is located behind the treatment, priority and filtering of incoming stimuli from our minds. The network is involved to produce these impressions and take decision on the measures that should be carried out.

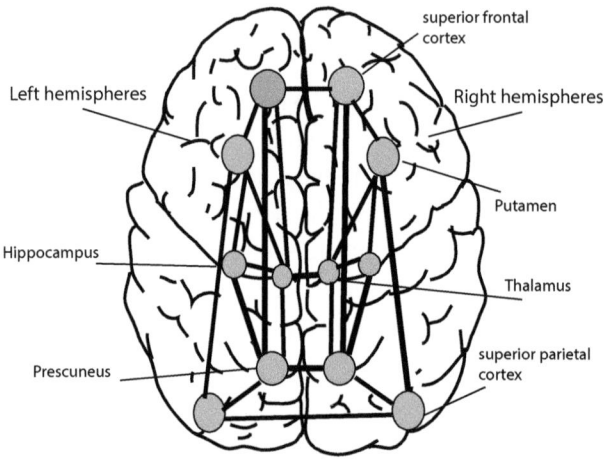

Fig. 1.13 Simplifyed figure of "rich club".

In a recent research reports by 2013 have scientists examined 41 schizophrenic patients for to see differences in "rich club" network in comparison with healthy volunteers (see ref. 1.19). The results showed that this group of schizophrenic patients has a reduction relating to nerve signals in these net-works. As a result, schizophrenic patients have a lower global capacity-functionality in "rich club" network and a different dynamics in nerve signals. The further research on these networks can provide a deeper understanding about neurological disorders and may be able to resolve the binding problem.

This chapter has especially focused on describing how the development of the human nervous system and its neural delays impacting our ability to perceive "real world" now. The chapter also tries to provide a background to "the unconscious" different influences of our experiences, reactions and decisions in many situations in which we are unaware. In the following chapters, many of these properties are the basis of how we experience various influences such as e.g. intuition, body language and body consciousness. Chapter 2 sets out in more detail for our sensory input compared to the various super senses which can be found in the rest of the animal world.

As illustration of "qualia" is quoted a few stanzas from the Nobel Literature Prize winner Tomas Tranströmer works.

From the memories look me (1993): Within me I wear my earlier faces, that a tree has its year rings. It is the sum of them who is "I". The mirror sees only my latest face, I know all my earlier.

Out of the night vision (1970): Two truths are coming out to each other. A coming from within, a coming from outside and where they meet, have you a chance to see yourself.

Chapter 2 Mind's limits

Super senses

This chapter deals with the various senses in the human body that creates the experiences in the present. Human perception of the surrounding world is in principle restricted to the physical phenomena that our minds can register. We may for example perceiving some electromagnetic radiation field in limited areas as light waves (visible light wavelength approximately 400 - 780 nanometers), heat waves, but not other kinds of electromagnetic fields such as shortwave radio, radar pulses, x-ray or nuclear radiation. These types of radiation to which we are not consciously aware for example microwaves, UV light or x-ray waves is dangerous for man and can , among other things cause damage to the eyes or cause future cancer diseases. Therefore, there are limits for these types of radiation that responsible authorities created to prevent people not are exposed to these kinds of harmful radiation (see figure 2.1).

In the chapter will respective mind to be described and it's limited regarding for example the minimum sound pressure to be able to hear the faintest sounds (the coverage threshold). Under the heading super senses refers to comparisons with other species to show the difference compared to human level of sensitivity and scope in the different senses. Many of the published charts that display the properties of the human senses represent usually averages in a larger population, while individuals can have large variations in sensitivity to a particular mind. It will also be given some examples of exceptional skills where persons with e.g. Savant syndrome can have a huge memory capacity despite its other handicap. People with synesthesia can associate for example letters, words or days of the week associated with color experience. The limits are therefore different both people between and among different species. Where our human consciousness perceives a hot summer meadow in sunlight, a bee that has senses of ultraviolet light can see something completely different or a dog to experience an entire fragrance landscape.

As we saw in the previous chapter, it is man's central and peripheral nervous system that receives and processes all incoming stimuli from the environment. There is also the internal sense which regulates all the body's internal organ which is the prerequisite for our survival. One can roughly distinguish about twenty-seven different senses (receptors) which supply the central nervous system with information on many predictors in the body like temperature, body position, hydration, bowel function and any damages, etc.

The internal environment in the body is controlled in high degree of the autonomic nerve system, that we are not normally aware of. This system has a number of receptors which keeps the body in an inner balance by, among other things the hypothalamus controls thirst from sensors for hydration, the brainstem has receptors for blood sugar levels and PH-value, the lungs have reached sensitive receptors of air flow that controls breathing, urine function has reached the sensitive receptors in the bladder and stretch receptors in the stomach and bowel for regulation of hunger. Some of these unconscious autonomous functions can by training been control mentally, where for example Yoga exercises can affect breathing rate and heart rhythm. You can even control the metabolism of the body so that lethargy of consciousness is achieved.

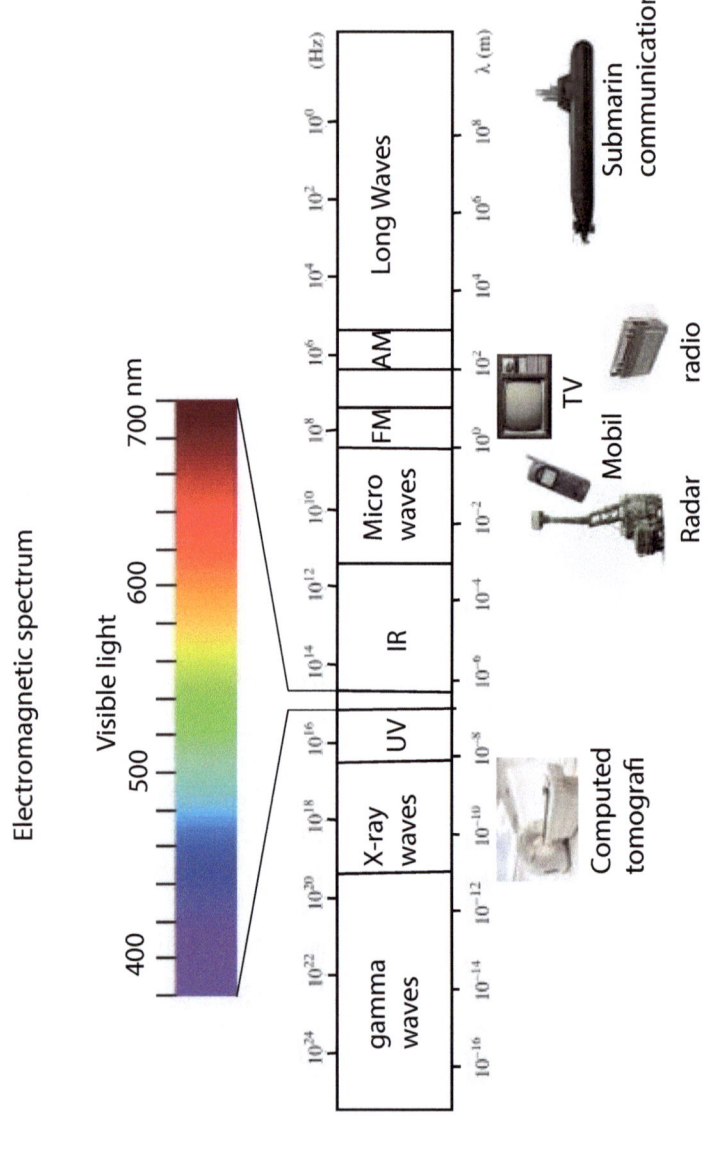

Electromagnetic spectrum

Visible light

400 500 600 700 nm

gamma waves	X-ray waves	UV	IR	Micro waves	FM	AM	Long Waves	
10^{24}	10^{22}	10^{20}	10^{18}	10^{16}	10^{14}	10^{12}	10^{10}	10^{8}	10^{6}	10^{4}	10^{2}	10^{0} (Hz)
10^{-16}	10^{-14}	10^{-12}	10^{-10}	10^{-8}	10^{-6}	10^{-4}	10^{-2}	10^{0}	10^{2}	10^{4}	10^{6}	10^{8}	λ (m)

Computed tomografi

Radar

Mobil

TV

radio

Submarin communication

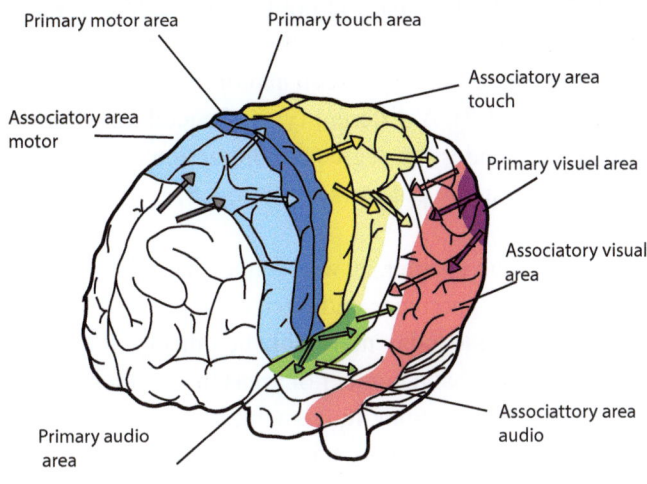

Fig. 2.2 cortex anatomy, primary och associatory areas.

When it comes to the external environment mentions it usually that man has the five senses sight, hearing, touch, smell and taste. But if you look to the involved receptors can be grossly increase the number to nineteen. In your eyes we have two types of receptors rods and cones, the sense of smell has on the one hand, a large number of olfactory receptors and partly an organ for pheromones, in taste the mind can discern five different tastes, skin tactile mind has seven different receptors, sense of balance is basalt for how we can go and body mind which contains a number of proprioceptors are constantly working out where we have our limbs.

How the mind perceives the stimuli from the different senses are affected by a number of elements, where perception and its constitution is coded in the brain and nervous system in various ways. You can start with a first way of a pressure-sensitive thatch in the hand through the press gives a way a signal in a pressure-sensitive receptor. The stimulus provides a pulse action of nerve that via spinal cord is passed to the primary somatosensory cortex in the brain. For that the brain must be able to know the origin of a nerve signal have the evolution created the primary somatosensory area in the cortex where each nerve cell anatomically represents its place in the body (see figure 1.7). A different type of encoding is for example when a motor neuron encodes the degree of contraction in a muscle via to increase the frequency of nerve pulses (see figure 1.6).

In the previous chapter, it was found that when it comes to how the mind receives its experience and interpretation of such as sights (the binding problem) there is today no established theory. Research on how sights shaped, has shown that a number of areas in the cerebral cortex is involved in the interpretation of color, movement, location and recognition of visual objects. According to a theory can synchronized oscillations between different clusters of nerve cells communicate common perceptual expression through the neural networks. In this context, it may be interesting to a concept created by professors Christof Koch and Francis Crick (The neuronal correlates of consciousness, NCC) which involves the definition of the minimum presence of a neural event and mechanism that together form a specific perception (experience) see Ref. 2.1.

In the brain's anatomy can be distinguished primary areas in the cortex where the sensory nerve signals (movement, sense of touch, sight and hearing) are received in the central nervous system (CNS) and where a first primary analysis of incoming stimuli are made (see fig. 2.2). Adjacent to the primary areas are a secondary association area for every mind where a refined analysis of the processed signal is made for that shape a perception of the experience. Cortex outside these areas is associative areas which are involved in the complex higher mental processes such as language ability, thinking, planning and doing coordination (integration) between the different sensory sensations. For language ability can, for example have the input from the different senses like sight (reading of books), tactile (Braille, alphabet for the blind) or via your hearing. The following covers a description of the different senses with a deeper review of the sense of sight then this is most explored and can work as a general description of the mechanisms in the cortex basic functions.

We have for the different senses measured up the minimum activity by stimuli for that perceived by the conscious mind. For e.g. hearing has the coverage threshold, the conscious strength (amplitude) and frequency range within which the sound can be understood measured up. When it comes to the content of the information in our various minds are the visual cues that are dominant with inflowing of ca 10 Mbit/s (10000000 bits per second) to the brain's visual cortex. The processing of this huge amount of information requires about 50% of calculation power in the brain and this reflected if you measure the EEG signals. When you have closed eyes dominate alpha waves (8-13 Hz) but as soon as your eyes opened may to a dominance of beta waves (about 13- 40 Hz) which characterizes conscious alertness. Total inflow of information from the senses is about 11 Mbit/s where touch generates about 1 Mbit/s, hearing 100 Kbit/s, smell 100 Kbit/s and taste about 1 Kbit/s. This large amount of input can consciousness not handle way different support centers in the cortex takes care of detective-adjustment, classification and compilation of these data. Only max display order about 40 bit/s is presented for conscious evaluation.

Sense of sight

You can say that when it comes to the sense of sight is the retinal light-sensitive retina at the rear side of the eyes the bottom central and can be seen as a part of the brain's visual structure. The kind of eyes that humans and primates have can be likened to a camera's eye where you behind the cornea have a lens that show an up and down image of the surroundings on the retina like a camera's way to expose a film. Retinal structure is extremely complex with about 10 layers of light-sensitive neurons and ganglia cells for registration of luminous flux and color.

In each eye retina are about 130 million neurons that are sensitive to blue-white light called rods and about 7 million nerve cells of three different types called cones that are sensitive to red, green and blue light. Throw to mix the three base color like red, green and blue, you can obtain all the different colors in the visible spectrum. These total 137 million neuronal signals are encoded in order to be able to be transferred to the brain's visual cortex via the optic nerve which contains approximately 1 million nerve paths. Recently has discovered another type of light-sensitive retinal ganglia cells which only reacts to blue light which has a own nerve path, that sends signals to a collection of cells in the brain which is called suprachiasmatic core. This center acts as the body's "the clock" and shuts down the production of melatonin during the light time of the day.

Distribution of rods and cones are uneven where the 7 million color sensitive cones are centered in the fovea and the so called yellow spot centrally placed in the eye's focal point, while the 130 million rods are spaced along the rest of the retina in figure 2.3. A different function in the eye's anatomy is that the rods away from the fovea has been combined into larger receptive fields than for the cones that have small receptive fields which also meant that visual acuity is lower in the peripheral areas of the retina. You could say that the rods which are the order of 1000 times more sensitive for light than cones works in low light at night without color and cones are active in normal daylight and generate our view of color. As shown in the picture, there is an area about 15 degrees from the fovea in the retina where the optic nerve to the brain goes out from the eye and there is a lack of light receptors why it is called "blind spot". Normally we not see this blind spot because the both eyes came to complement each other in the visual brain function and also when we see with one eye fills the brain out this area with nearby sights.

A way to self-experience the blind spot is to turn the left eye off and fix his gaze on the top of the outstretched left thumb with your right eye. Move slowly it stretched index finger on right hand at arm's length from right up the left thumb with eye fixed on it. We see then that the right index finger disappears from the peripheral field of view when your fingers are about 15 - 25 cm apart corresponding to the 15 degrees as the blind spot is displaced from the fovea. While moving within 5 degrees in this position, it is impossible to perceive right index finger.

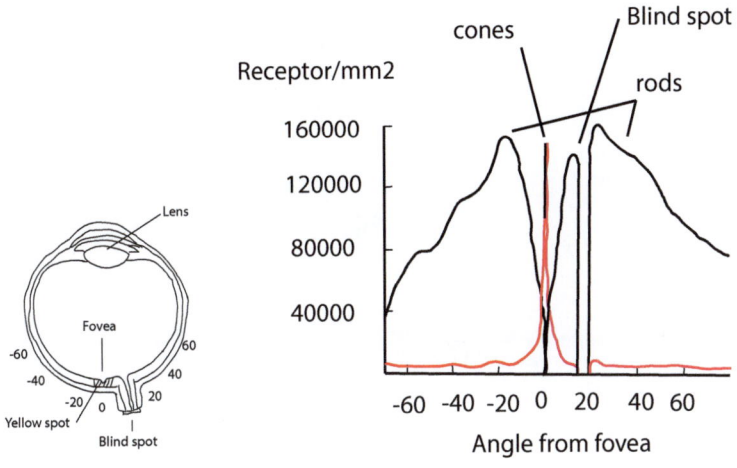

Fig. 2.3 Eyes anatomy and receptors.

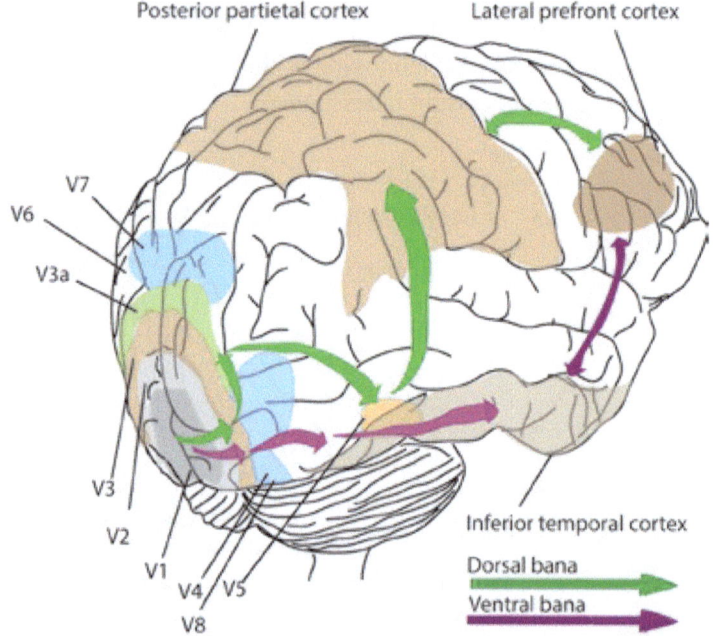

Figur 2.4 Area för visual information

On the basis of that eye's focus point is located in the yellow spot is it where the sharpening is greatest while it decrease along the rest of the retina. In order to get a sharp image has eye 6 different muscles controlled by the brain's visual function so that if we for example read the text in a book is done automatic unconscious eyes movement (called saccades) which gradually focuses the eye on the read text. These muscles is also governed by our balance system to stabilize the sight in movements of the head when otherwise a jumping experience of the field of view would be like when a watching of a video taken with hand mobile camera. In order to stabilize the image, there is a automatic mechanisms in the brain's visual cortex that compensates for when your eyes blink quickly for example between the fix points that the eye takes in the reading of a line of text.

Optic nerves from each eye are shared so that the left field of vision in each eye goes to the right hemisphere visual cortex while the right vision field goes to the left hemisphere visual cortex. This means that each eye views the nerve from the nose side of the retina is crossover between the cerebral hemispheres. Further goes sight nerves through a structure in the thalamus called the lateral geniculate nucleus (LGN) and brought forward to the visual cortex, which is located at the rear against the neck. LGN has, among other things a function for analysis of time dependency between different sights and can focus on what that is important in a visual signal. If you for example hear a sound in the environment gives signals from hearing to the LGN task about where the eyes should be directed to that regard the area from whence the sound came.

The area where visual cues from the LGN are processed further called primary visual cortex or abbreviated V1 then this structure was the first area in the mapping of vision. Then have a number of additional functional areas for visual processing identified what is termed V2, V3, V4, V5, V6, V7 and V8. These different areas are organized in different ways for example left and right-eye neurons are varied in parallel layers. The mapping and original title of these visual centers emanates from in-depth studies of the monkey macaques on which much research has been carried out through direct measurement of nerve signals in the visual cortex and visual perception have been mapped in detail.

When it comes to the human brain is that during the last few decades it has had the opportunity to study visual centers with PET, fMRI and MEG equipment that researcher started to map out the details in the brain's processing of visual input. The Names V1... V8 from macaques have also been applied to the corresponding visual areas in the human brain, but in the literature are also a number of alternative names. Then it in this presentation just made a rough description of the function the different visual field in treatment of sights wills only these designations to be used.

The researchers who works in the visual area of the brain is not completely agree on the main function of each center in visual perception but the following description gives a picture of current research results. In the following is accounted for each visual area in the brain with the description of the main function and even where it is relevant what problems that occur in a patient if the area is damaged for example by stroke. Figure 2.4 shows the approximate location of the respective areas.

V1: The primary visual cortex is in principle an area with neurons whose inputs come through LGN from the cells of the retina and can be said to reflect a certain point in the field of view for each neuron. When the number of view cells in the fovea and yellow stain has the largest resolution is the corresponding area in the V1 most of that and decline to the outside edges. In addition, the processed signals from cones and rods are not in the same structure but are differenced. V1 make easier treatment of sights, e.g. do detective-orientation of edges between black and white fields and decoding brightness. Damage to V1 shows up directly in the field of view of e.g. a stroke damaged patient through dark fields in each field of view.

V2: Next Visual area called V2 and is the first in a number of associative areas that receive their input from V1 but give also feedback back to V1. V2 passes visual information to areas V3, V4 and V5 and is involved in the detection of complex couture, stereoscopic vision, illusive detection of shapes and distinguish shapes from the background.

V3/V3a: Register angles and symmetries and are involved at be act of global movement.

V4/V8: V4 is an area that is affected strongly when we give attention to something in the field of view. The area is involved for color detection but also participates in the orientation and spatial perception. Later research with fMRI points out the neighboring area V8 as the most focused area of color detection. Damage from stroke can in these areas lead to total color blindness (Achromatopsia) which gives a black and white experience of the environment.

V5: Is a visual area with many relations both with V1, V2, V3 and other areas of the cortex and is mainly involved in the perception of movement and binocular vision. The area detects movement, movement speed, detection of stereoscopic depth and control of range of eye movement. Damage in this area means that the patient cannot see movement (akinetopsia), which give a problem for example when you put coffee in a cup or do not see vehicle movement at the intersection of a street because he seeing the world in separated images.

V6: Is associated with its own motion and peripheral vision. It includes an area with topographical oriented visual field of the surroundings and has a high specificity for orientation of edges.

V7: deals with the perception of symmetry.

These parallel visual centers are focused on various properties, such as color, shape, size, movement, and orientation of visual information and results in the picture as the mind seeing. How the brain coordinates all these brain areas called "the binding problem" is not completely charted.

Two researchers L G Ungerleider and M Mishkin at the National Institute of Mental Health Washington D.C. who researched on monkeys visual cortex published a report in 1982 (ref. 2.2) in which it suggested that the visual information followed two different cortical pathways where associative data processing took place partly in the posterior parietal cortex (PP) on the issue "was" the visual image is, while the question " What " image represents are treated in a cortical circuit in inferior temporal cortex (IT), see figure 2.4. In the dorsal ride from visual cortex to PP treated the spatial parameters that an object's location in relation to a person and handles even information over a plan how for example the motoric must be controlled and timing to hold of a glass. Much of this control of motor function is completely unconscious and brought forward to the association areas of the prefrontal lobe, where a center for planning of movement is located, see figure 2.4. Damage from such as stroke in the dorsal path in a patient may cause difficulty in grasping a glass then the spatial perception is disturbed.

The ventral surface, "what", goes from the visual cortex through IT where the correlation looks made against previous visual memories for to identify the object's shapes or facial recognition. Even emotional information in the image can be conveyed to the amygdala, which is involved in the detection of possible fear situations. The result is transmitted on to the frontal lobe, where a perceptually consciousness on picture occur, see figure 2.4. Damage in the ventral course where a specific area for facial recognition is available can result in difficulty to recognize even their closest friends' faces (prosopagnosia). It has been made measurements in this area, associated with brain surgery for epilepsy, and researchers have been able to identify the individual neurons that are activated by the images of a particular known person that e.g. president Bill Clinton and Hollywood actress Jennifer Aniston. We have given this type of nerve cell nicknamed "grandmother cell".

Intensive research is going on in the mapping of the human visual perception for solving the binding problem, and then it is likely that the visual perception in the brain works on similar manner as between the brain's several areas for treatment of other perception. In figure 2.5 shows a simplified flowchart of how the visual information from the eye's retina processes in the various visual centers. In this context , mention the concept of blind vision that means that people who are totally blind to because of damage to the primary visual cortex (V1) still can perceive specific visual information from the eye's retina, then about 10 % of visual nerve signals go to these other visual areas.

Researcher Professor in neuroscience at the Tilburg University in Holland Beatrice de Gelder has, among other things conducted experiments with blind people who have seen images with strong emotional content and via sensors in their facial muscles were able to detect similar facial expressions as shown on a monitor of the subject (see ref. 2.3). These experiments have shown that many visual stimuli as color, simple former, simple movement and orientation of objects have been singled out despite that the person would not have been able to see any visual image. This indicates that there are neural networks in addition to V1 that provides visual information to the different cortical visual centers.

Another property of the visual perception is when in your imagination envisions mental image in the visual cortex. Measurements with fMRI shows that the same associative visual areas involved in the visual tasks of imagined image as in this case in corresponding to external visual stimuli from the eyes. In the prefrontal lobe is the activation of these areas almost entirely identical to a corresponding external image. Even in the case of the parietal lobe is the same line. In the temporal lobe, which is involved in the storage of visual memories and can be activated by signals both from lower levels and higher levels in the cortical visual processes, on the other hand, a measurable difference in activation in the two cases are found.

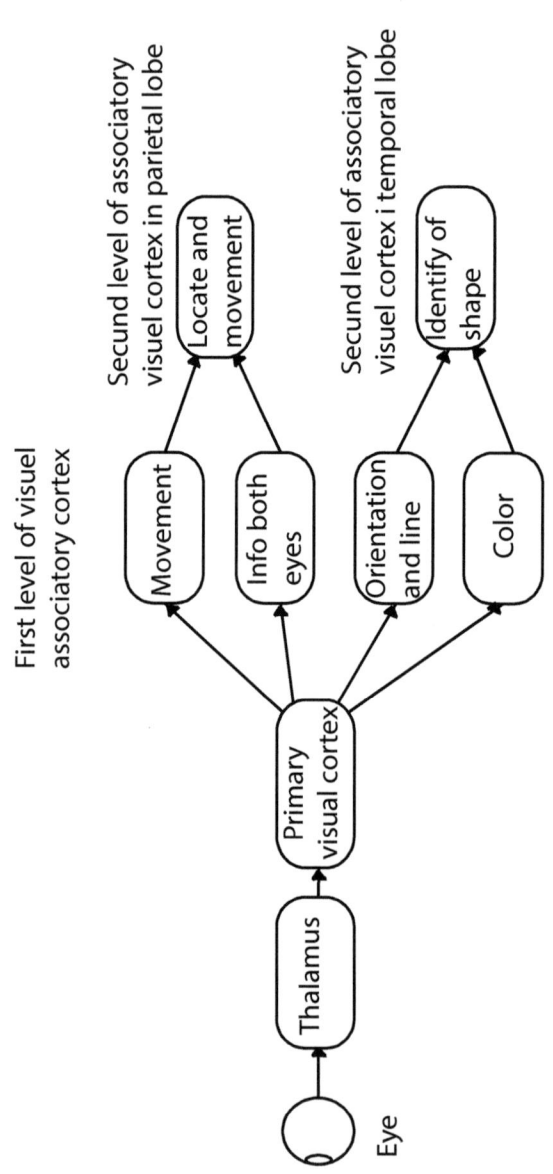

Fig. 2.5 Flow chart visual information.

Other experiments have shown on the plasticity that is available in the brain for learning of visual information. If a test subject to be fitted with glasses that provide a reverse picture of the outside world, he will in a matter of hours have become accustomed to this new perception and the visual centers have been able to reverse the perception so that an upright image perceived by the person. After one such experiment it takes a number of hours before the visual experience returns to normal function again.

When it comes to visual experiences there are ongoing research at Karolinska Institutet in Stockholm by Professor Henrik Ehrsson at the Department of neuroscience about how we as humans create our unconscious body consciousness. In order to create the illusion that a rubber arm that is on the table in front of the subject is the person›s own need to two senses that are synchronized in a common experience. The subject sits at a table where for example the left arm is hidden behind a screen while a rubber arm at the bottom of the screen is visible to the subject. By touching both the left arm and rubber arm at the same time, to get volunteers to experience the rubber arm as a part of the body and if you suddenly hit with a hammer on the rubber arm reacts the subject awesome then rubber arm has taken a position in the subject›s knowledge. Through the use of fMRI equipment have it been able to map out the centers of the brain as in this case, connect the visual image with the tactile touch.

At last for the visual perception is given some examples of limit values for the sense of sight and comparison with the animal world›s super senses. In terms of visual acuity, the ability to distinguish small details in view-field is defined by to test how close two small points can approach each other before they are perceived as a single and is referred to as resolution capability. Visual acuity is matched by the angle where you still see two points. It specifies the visual acuity with a number for example 1.0 or 0.5 and value 1.0 which is common in healthy people is the equivalent of a point of view on 1 minute of arc. Visual acuity varies both among different individuals and is also affected by the aging process. Many young people tend to have a better visual acuity within the range of 1.3 - 1.5 and it found single individuals with a visual acuity at 2.0 and the highest measured is around 2.3. In the animal world are the Raptors who have the sharpest sight with two yellow spots as a concave dimple in the retina which gives an effect as a telephoto lens that magnifies the sharp image. An Eagle have approximately 5 times more light-sensitive cells than a human being and a Golden Eagle can perceive small movements of a rabbit on more than two kilometers distance, according to the Guinness Book of animal records.

In terms of light sensitivity are the rods about 1000 times more sensitive to light than the cones and gives black and white vision at night. In the animal world is the owl that has best night vision which is about 100 times better than a human›s eyes. First, the owl tubular eyes, can broaden the pupils maximum and has a highly tissue layer behind the retina that enhances the light to the retina.

Human sight of color differs from many animal ways to see the light spectrum. Many mammals such as e.g. dogs and squirrels have only two types of cones (dichromatic) while the man has three types of cones (trichromatic). There are exceptions where about 10 % of women have an inherited change in the retina with four types of cones for sight of color (tetra chromatic). At normally sight of color (trichromatic) man expect to be able to discern about 10 million shades of colors while a woman with tetra chromatic sight of color can distinguish 10 times more shades (about 100 millions). About 10 percent of the male population have defects in their sight of color due to inherited defects in the single x chromosome, which means that the person often confuse red and green. Birds have the well-developed sight of color with five different color receptors combined with five different filters in the retina. A curiosity in this context is that the perception of color can vary between different nations dependent on linguistic or cultural differ. Fore example in the English language world defines 8 different basic colors (red, orange, green, blue, purpura, yellow, brown and black) while one of the indigenous people of New Guinea had five categories of colors.

Humans have with the single exception no vision in UV and infrared areas while many animals are specialized to see within these frequency ranges. Some snakes has nose organ which is sensitive to infrared radiation and are aware of the changes in total darkness while for example bee has a capacity to see UV-light which guides to blossom nectar. Another feature is the light adaption in the eyes of a human being makes to flashing images with higher frequency than about 16 frames per second seems to be moving while an insect can perceive up to 300 frames per second. This allows our 50 Hz electricity networks perceived give flashing lights for a fly. The Sun›s rays vibrate normally in all plans but in earth›s atmosphere affects the light to become polarized, giving a pattern in the sky which shows the Sun›s location. Bees use this polarized light on cloudy days to locate the path to the hive.

The sense of hearing

Human hearing is designed to receive signals which are transmitted via the pressure fluctuations in air or via vibrations in solid structures and the rise of with so called longitudinal waves. This in contrast to electro-magnetic waves which are transverse propagation (waves perpendicular to direction of motion). The ear is classified in the three zones external pinnae, middle ear and the inner ear (see figure 2.6). The outer ear is designed to absorb sound waves and they are led through the ear canal to the eardrum that is set in vibration as sound waves. Eardrum lining is bulkhead between external pinnae and middle ear where the three bone hammer, anvil, and stirrup transmits the pressure waves on to further a film that is called the oval window. The Oval window conveys the variety in pressure to the cochlea.

The difference between the larger drum of the womb area and oval window›s area results in a strengthening of the pressure in the audio signal at about 15 times , which is conveyed to the fluid-filled cochlea. Structure of the cochlea is similar to form a spiral shaped sea shells and is inside the split in two about 3 cm long channels shared by a membrane (basilar membrane) on which hair cells are placed which gives signals to the auditory nerve. In the end of the cochlea is more a membrane which is called round window which is involved in the reflection of sound wave. When the liquid is put in oscillation by movements in the oval window, a wave of hearing cochlea liquid affecting the basilar membrane whereby sensory hairs provides information about frequency and amplitude on the received audio. The audio signal is transmitted further via the auditory nerve to the primary auditory cortex.

Hair cells in basilar membrane sitting in groups along the cochlea spiral where those that are sensitive to high tones are closest to the oval window and low tones recorded at the far end of the membrane (called a tonotopy order). Auditory nerve for each frequency goes to the primary auditory cortex where the receiving neurons are localized in a similar way in a rising rate scale.

There are two interpretations how auditory signals detected of which one is called place theory. Place theory specifies that the sound signal frequency causing a stimulus of the hair cells via its location on basilar membrane for a specific frequency. The second method called the periodicity theory which indicates that the cortex interprets the sound with respect to the periodicity of nerve action potential signals. Current theories believe that higher frequencies are interpreted according to place theory while detection of bass frequencies is performed with periodicity theory. Auditory nerves from the right and the left ear is like many other senses crossover to the opposite hemisphere, but there is also a part of the auditory nerve which is attached to the same hemisphere in the brain.

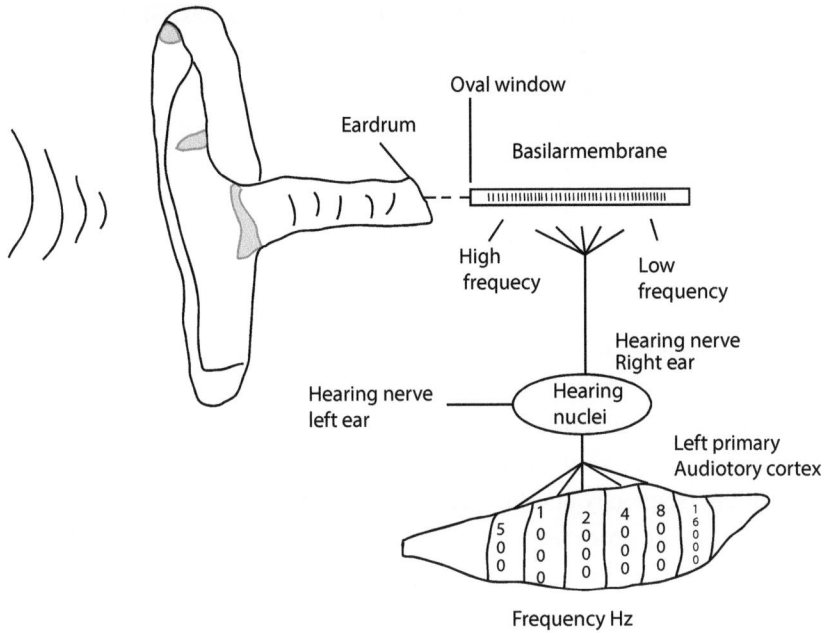

Fig. 2.6 Ear and cochlea

Before the audio signal going to the primary auditory cortex the signal is processed in a number of centers including: in the thalamus, which acts as a relay station for detection of time, frequency and spatial information. The exact function of each of these nuclei are not completely known but the structure with tonotopy order of signals and the thesis is binaural listening (locate from where the sound is coming) is maintained, among other things. Signals from both ears are compared for perception of time differences and density modulation between the audio signals.

Some of these grains and their main function are described below.

• Cochlear nuclei: contains neurons that react on a ton beginning, others react continuously; others react to fast frequency or intensity modulation.

• Superior olive: Is bilateral mix by input from the right and left ear. Coding of audio in relation to where they came from.

• Inferior colliculus: Have two way communications with auditory cortex. It is sensitive to time and spatial change and binaural stimulation.

Primary hearing cortex is located in the temporal lobe of cortex (see fig. 2.2) and is involved in basic detection of for example music by interpretation of the frequency and loudness. The surrounding secondary associative auditory cortex processes the harmonic, melodic and rhythmic patterns in the sound. When it comes to speaking, there are two alleged cortical areas that have specific features in language understanding, of which the one called Wernicke's area which is involved in the understanding of spoken and written language while Brocas area controls how the spoken word is generated.

It has mapped out the human hearing by measuring how the ear perceives the weakest sound level (the coverage threshold) and how the ear perceives different frequencies in the sound. Depends on the shape design and the hearing bone conveys sound signal sound pressure to the oval window showing measurements that the ear is most sensitive between 3000 Hz to 4000 Hz (see figure 2.7). The coverage threshold is set at 2000 Hz at a sound pressure on $p0 = 20$ µPa (0.00002 N/m2). As the lower tone curve in figure 2.7 shows required much stronger signal in the lower frequency ranges to originate the same sound pressure at 1000 Hz. The ear perception of different sound levels follows a logarithmic scale of sound pressure is expressed as , $SPL = 10 \cdot LOG10 (p/p0) 2$ [dB], " sound pressure level (SPL) ", where 10 logarithm of expression define the measuring value in dB . The diagram shows that the ear can manage a large dynamic range from 0 dB at 1000 Hz up to about 120 dB. At about 140 dB reaches the ear a pain threshold where hearing is exposed to serious damage causing future hearing problems.

At measurement of sound levels in the context of e.g. noise investigations from traffic or train traffic uses to filter weighing that mimics the frequency dependence and these filters are designated A, B or C and specified in with measured noise level for example 80 dB (A). Ear's frequency response is often cited as 20 -20000 Hz which applies for young people, then especially the high frequency range is affected by age for that at 60 years of age has dropped to about
10 KHz. For speaking play this not so great part where it counts with 300-3400 Hz to be able to perceive speech with good quality.

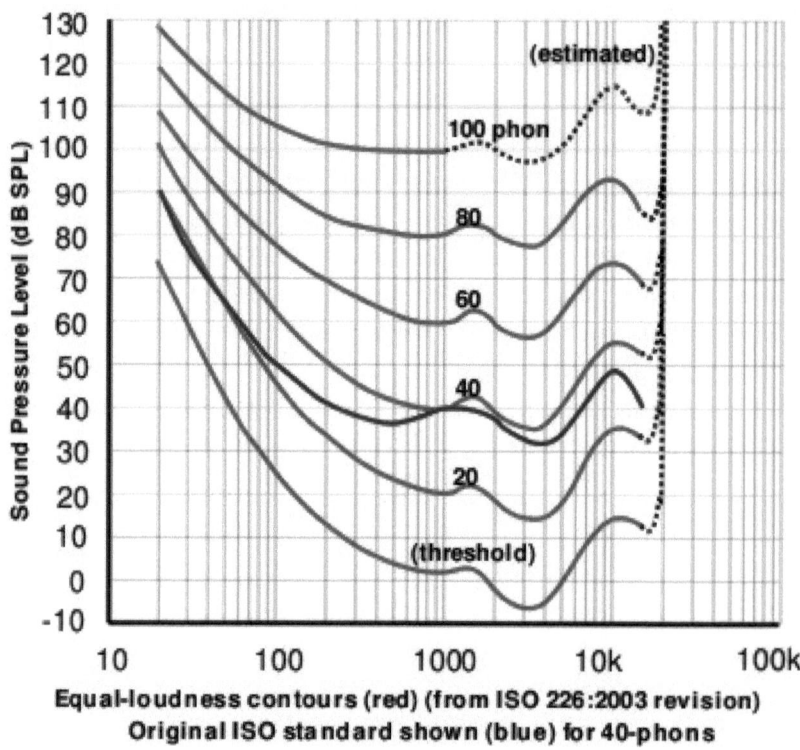

Equal-loudness contours (red) (from ISO 226:2003 revision)
Original ISO standard shown (blue) for 40-phons

Fig. 2.7 Frequency curves and the coverage threshold. From wikipedia (http://en.wikipedia.org/wiki/Equal-loudness_contour).

In the associative areas of auditory cortex, there is a number of abilities that characterize the hearing there, for example has the ability to focus on an interesting conversation in the presence of high background noise. You can also by binaural listening quite exactly point out where a sound source coming from. In the higher associative areas of the cortex are also coupling stations (PIPs) which creates connections between the senses so that for example a strong concern audio can enable eye movements to the sides and even emotionally affect the amygdala to put body in readiness for action. When it comes to the two brain hemispheres auditory cortex can you discern certain characteristics listed in table 2.1.

Left auditiva cortex	Right auditiva cortex
Analytic	Understand visuel presentation of word
Sequence	Process intonation pattern
Control speech	Recognize emotion prosodi
Discriminate language sound	Understand jokes
Preceive temporal rhythm	Process speech structure
Linear	Holistic

Table 2.1 Characteristics of auditory cortex left, right.

Broca area: Can lead to speaking not become liquid and without syntax.
Wernicke's area: Speak may be liquid but meaningless (nonsense).

Here are some examples of the limits when it comes to hearing for different animals. When it comes to the coverage threshold are desert dwelling animal often good hearing that for example muse who by the receptive structure has about 5 times better hearing of weak sounds and can be warned by the weak sound from a owl wings. Humans have a great capacity to determine where a sound is coming but for example tower owl can perceive a three dimensional map of sound. Tower owl have audio channel upward on the right side and downward on the left side so that the sound can also be located vertically.

When it comes to frequency ranges for example a dog hearing up to 40 KHz which, among other things utilized by the use of high-frequency whistles for to give command to the dog. Different mice use sounds up to 100 KHz for communication, but when a cat can hear up to 70 KHz are the most excellent mice hunters. Elephants have an organ in the pan that can generate infrasound below 10 Hz which is used for communication within a herd of elephants.

A different way to use the audio is bat way to use ultrasound for echo location. Through large hinged ear can bats send short sound pulses to the surroundings and listen to the echo pulses reflected from surrounding former. Through to vary the number of pulses per time-unit (from about 10 times/s up to 200 times/s) can a bat locate prey with great accuracy. The ultrasound can be produced up to 200 KHz and in some cases, the frequency during the sound pulse be varied in order to obtain better resolution. Some species also uses Doppler Effect to measure the speed and direction of travel for the target.

The sense of smell

The sense of smell, which is our oldest sense, is unlike other perception linked directly to the limbic system (sometimes referred to as the "reptilian brain") without passing through the thalamus. Typically, the sense of sight is given priority among the brain's sensory expressions with their often exact personal memories, while the sense of smell is a powerful and direct impact on the emotional area.

In his novel "in the search after the time that has gone" gives the writer Marcel Proust a vivid description of the childhood memories that are developed by the aroma from eating a madeleine cake dipped in tisane tee. These scent sticks brought the author back to his childhood where his aunt Leonie served these accessories before Sunday's show. Proust pointed out that these taste and olfactory memories has a strong impact on special children's flashbacks in which the scent from the mother and other experiences are stored as complete footprint and can be developed by second rapid scent string. A quote from the book gives a performance of these impact: " But then noting other remains of a transition time, when people have died and things destroyed, so liver even perfume and taste alone remains; fragile but viable, more intangible, more faithful and longer lasting. As the dead people's souls will take the even long left among the memories after all the others; they remember, remember, hope and carry that on an almost unsightly small water drops surface memory tremendous building".

Smell has a direct link to the amygdala, which is the brain's warning center for incoming threats from the senses, presents a direct connection in order to avoid the dangers from the route food or contaminated water.

The human sense of smell is a form of chemo reception where the odor receptor in the nose serves as complex molecule detectors. The odor receptors is placed within a stamp footprint area in the upper part of the nasal cavity and consists of a mucous membrane, olfactory epithelium, containing a variety of cell types including the olfactory receptor neuron, ORN, is most important. These receptors are embedded in the lining and have cilia for to capture the fragrant compounds, see fig. 2.8. Gaseous air particles must first resolve itself in mucus before the influence of odor receptors can be made. At a cold which provides inflammation in nasal mucosa loses it in the acute stage is often the smell and taste of food gone. When these receptors are continuously exposed to wear and tear through the air impact so live a odor cell ca 2 months before it is replaced.

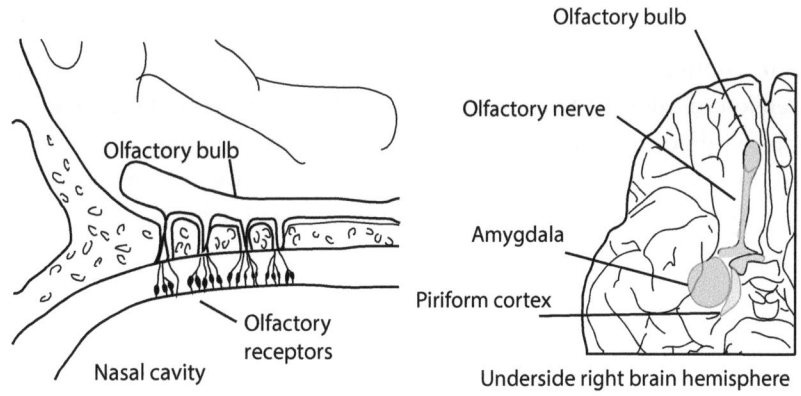

Fig. 2.8 Nasal cavity   Anatomy receptors

Humans have about 350 types of odor receptors that can discern different proteins and a total more than 10 million olfactory receptor neuron, ORN. The nasal mucosa is kept moist by secretions produced by glial cells that allow inhaled air to be moistened, is heated and provides a barrier that protects the lungs from infections.

The receptors for the same type of scents are connected in the olfactory bulb to cluster with up to 1000 cells before they are attached on to the olfactory nerve that conveys scent experience to the olfactory center in the temporal lobe of the cortex. In addition to the 350 types of odor receptors clean scent signal, patterns of several aroma receptors signal at the same time give 10000's of different compound fragrance experiencer. Later time research has pointed out that it is already in the nasal olfactory organ is a form of signal-processing in which different areas perceive pleasant or unpleasant smells that through the amygdala can trigger nausea at for example smell of rotten fish or trigger salivation in a mouthwatering scent.

In difference from other perception in the brain are olfactory nerves for each nostril connected directly to the same hemisphere›s olfactory centrum. Like that one for the sight and hearing can get stereoscopic information on the surrounding environment, can also smell feel of direction from were smells coming through by the difference between the two nasal cavitation detection of odor. At tests with outsourced odor trace on the ground have subjects blindfolded could follow odor trace by crawling and smell out there after the surface of the land. In figure 2.9 shows a schematic block diagram of how the olfactory information is spread in the brain›s olfactory areas.

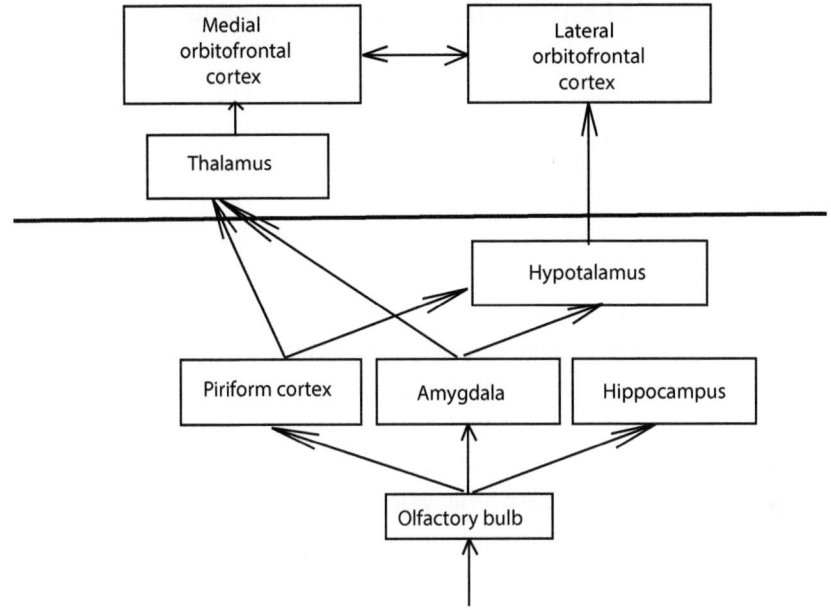

Fig. 2.9 Olfactory system

At the bottom of the schema will nerve impulses from ORN to olfactory bulb where a compendium of the various receptors 350 nerve signals are made for transport via first cranial nerve to the primary olfactory center in the temporal lobe. A part of the unconscious treatments of odor signals occurs in the amygdala, where any dangerous substances can give immediate spew symptom for to prevent ingestion. Storage of scent memories takes place through the hippocampus, which among other things are involved in long term storage of autobiographical or episodic memories which often includes location information, smell, taste, sight and hearing memories. Hippocampus manages the coordination of these memory fragments which are stored in various places in the cortex and recalled in the respective peace center at reactivation of memory. At storage of smell memories are also the emotional aspect involved which enable rewards center or evokes disgust against unpleasant scent. Piriform cortex can detect pheromones which can affect the hypothalamus handling of hormones that enable the interest in sexual signals from the opposite sex. On the conscious level is the orbitofrontal cortex in the frontal lobe, where the scents reaches a conscious level and can affect aware a person reaction on olfactory information

Within the animal values are an organ called vomeroasal organ which is located between the nose and the mouth. This organ is used in animal perception of pheromones which control much of animal behavior, in conjunction with pair bonding and reproduction. When it comes to human beings is too unsure on whether a corresponding organ is active when it is both underdeveloped or absent in some human. On the other hand, plays the endogenous substances pheromones are secreted in sweat and urine (which contains fragrances that tells us about sex, ovulation, immune defense, etc.) play a role in the same way in pair production and reproduction in humans. Pheromones are a flavorless substance that triggers nerve signals to a different part of the brain with a more bodily reaction than odor experience. Pheromones plays role in a flock or between different individuals of different sex and research has shown that for example women at the same workplace often synchronize their menstrual period. Women also have generally a better ability to smell than men. Hetero sexual women, for example activate the anterior hypothalamus (hormonal influence) by smell the derivatives of the male sex hormone and corresponding happens when men smell the female sex hormone. When it comes to partner selection have the immune system a major role where women prefer men who have a genotype of human leukocyte antigen (MHC) different from their own. Women who use oral contraceptives are affected so that they prefer MHC genotype similar to their own and get preference for feminine faces while women who do not eat the pill usually prefer masculine faces.

As for vision and hearing have researcher measured up and defined a number of parameters that quantify the measurement of human sensitivity to smell. Odors can be objectively evaluated through instrument olfactory meter which mixes the external air with col-filtered air. The instrument has a mouthpiece against respiratory and concentration-to-threshold monitoring is used by to increase the concentration of pure air until the subject does not consciously can perceive a smell. By measuring EEG signals on a subject, one can see that the brain reacts to lower concentrations of smells even before the person becomes aware of the smell. It is also a mechanism of habituation against an odor which the conscious experience of food is taken and may even disappear even though the smell cells continues send nerve impulse.

Presented below are some parameters that are commonly used for definition of the smell and the concentrations that could cause discomfort or injury in the lungs.

• Threshold in odor detection: the lowest concentration of smell detection.

• Detection of odor: Lowest concentration of odor identification.

• Intolerance of odor: Lowest concentration where the odor is dangerous or unacceptable.

• Sensory irritation: Lowest concentration where odor causing burning, irritating sensation.

It is for example rules from the WHO against harmful concentrations of odors that are based on responses from unease in a middle time of 30 minutes exposure. Large variations are available when it comes to the threshold of detection of such as substance hydrogen sulfide which is in the range 0.2-2.0 µg/m3, recognition 0.6-6.0 µg/m3 and guideline 7µg/m3. While the threshold for tetrachloroethylene is 1000 times higher with detection at 8 mg/m3, recognition 24-32 mg/m3 and benchmark 8 mg/m3.

General have man best odor sense in childhood which is reflected in the often intense scent memories that we have from childhood experiences. The ability to detect faint smells decline with age among according to gradually lose receptors in the nasal olfactory epithelium and bulb in the olfactory system. Presented below are some forms of neuroglial diseases of the olfactory system:

- Anosmia: Total lack of odor.

- Dysosmi: Smell memories are different from the current smell.

- Hyperosmi: Reduced sensitivity to smell.

- Hyposmia: Hypersensitivity to smells.

- Parosmia: Scents are perceived as unpleasant.

- Phantosmi: Hallucinatory odor often unpleasant.

Research when it comes to dementias like Alzheimer's and Parkinson's disease has discovered that the sense of smell in these diseases is significantly affected. The Director of the smell and taste research at the University of Pennsylvania Medical Center Richard L Doty who researched among others on Alzheimer's patients believes that you probably can detect precursors to Alzheimer's medical judgment by that test patients in an early stage. Proposal is to introduce routine odor test in connection with investigations of Alzheimer's disease.

In the animal world plays scents and pheromones a very major role in animal behavior under different season's conditions. During mating and rutting causes pheromones for sexual desire a great excitement of for example moose and deer which leads to bloody battles on female favor. Other mechanism are for example dogs and cats which urines to excel the own territory. If alien cats make intrusion on a cat's inner turf waged noisy cat fights especially during mating season.

In the case of sensitivity to fragrances is a man long after dogs tracking ability. If you compare the number of olfactory receptors for human ca 10-12 million odor cells, so have a regular dog about 1000 million cells and a bloodhound up to 4000 million cells. This reflects the large fragrance landscape as a dog experiences and the huge track susceptibility of a bloodhound. When it comes to insects so has research in the United States about the little black wasp "Microplitis Croceipes" taken science to a new level. Normally stings this wasp not people but use stinger to lay their eggs in the larvae to form the wasp larvae food supply. By these wasps have a sense of smell at the level of blood hounds can by training with the conditioned reflex can they be used instead of bomb dogs, or drug dogs. According to entomologist Joe Lewis at the University of Georgia, it only takes five minutes to work out the wasps. The hungry wasps may smell, for example a dead human body while getting eating sugar water in 10 seconds. After one minute is the procedure repeated and after three trainings interval associate the wasp the smell of food. Wasps stopped in a plastic container with a fan in one end called "Wasp Hound". Inside the container is a web camera that monitors five wasps and when wasps feel the smell the contingent gathered around the fan and thus pointing out a odor target. Wasps can work up to 48 hours at a stretch. Scientists believe that wasps or other insects can be searched by explosives on airports, find dead bodies or detect diseases in patients ' exhaled air. Vid other universities in United States have been trained to look for mines.

The sense of taste

The human sense of taste is the least developed of the mind, where it is primarily via the taste buds of the tongue and mouth can identify the five basic tastes of sweet, salty, sour, bitter and umami. The taste umami is a taste of meat which, among other things governed by the amino acid glutamate, which is included in the meat, fish and stored cheese. The overall experience at the ingestion of food includes taste, smell and tactile information, where the smell often makes up 80-90 % of the unique experience (flavor). The taste receptors are like the olfactory receptors for smell a form of chemo receptors that are sensitive to substances dissolved in saliva. The different types of receptors located in bedded in the taste buds with finger like offshoots called microvilli can identify the specific receptor molecules for each of the topics concerned with food see fig. 2.9. It also includes filamentous papillae which does not contain taste receptors but is linked to the somatosensory cortex of detection of texture, temperature and consistency.

More recent research has indicated that there is about 30 different receptors for taste bitter that can give a complex taste experience. It is also a genetic influence when it comes to taste for bitter where 2/3 of the population know the topics 6-n-propylthiouracil (PROP) and phenylthiocarbamide (PTC) as much bitter while the other 1/3 part know very little of these tastes. Then taste cells in the tongue as well as scent cells in the nasal epithelium is exposed to abrasion, in the case of chewing of food, they are replaced every 10 days. Taste cells called papillae are small lumpy or pleated formations spread out on the tongue, the palate and in the pharynx and contains taste cells where each receptor cell is sensitive to several different flavors. A human being has approximately 5,000-10,000 taste buds scattered throughout the tongue surface layer and each taste bud contains about 50-70 receptor cells.

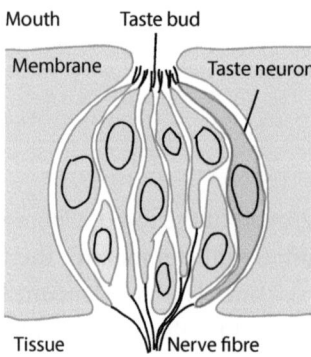

Fig. 2.9 Principled image taste buds .

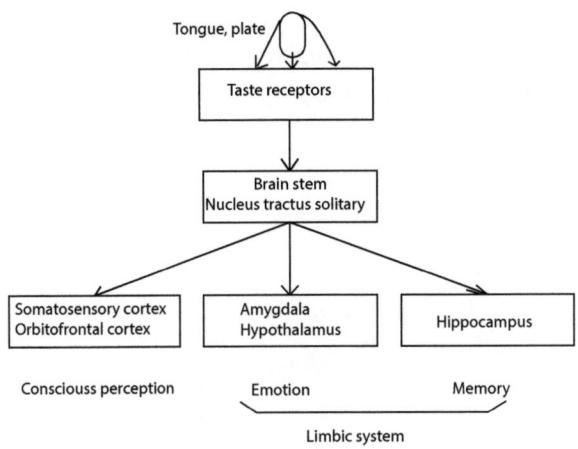

Fig. 2.10 Brain taste areas.

Nerve signals from the tongue and mouth goes through three different cranial nerve connections to the brain, where the front tongue goes via the facial nerve, posterior tongue goes to swallow nerve while the mouth goes via valgus nerve. Taste signals are processed in several different centers in the brain (see fig. 2.10, 2.11).

According to the figure go taste nerves via two different neural routes partly to the limbic system (amygdala, hippocampus and hypothalamus) where emotional reactions regarding the food appetite, aversion or maybe nostalgic feelings are activated and partly through the thalamus to the cerebral cortex in which different areas detects food's taste and tactile properties and that makes taste sensation awareness. The primary way for nerve signals are first to nuclei in the brainstem (nucleus tractus solitaire) then to the thalamus for further promotion to primary taste center (Insula) in addition to the somatosensory cortex, amygdala, orbitofrontal cortex hippocampus and hypothalamus.

In primary taste center is identification of taste and its intensity. The first sensations from your mouth are interpreted in the primary taste center with information about texture, temperature and similar tactile information. After about 200 milliseconds there is information on taste quality to be identified. After approximately 1 second there is information if the food is dangerous or unpleasant to be extracted.

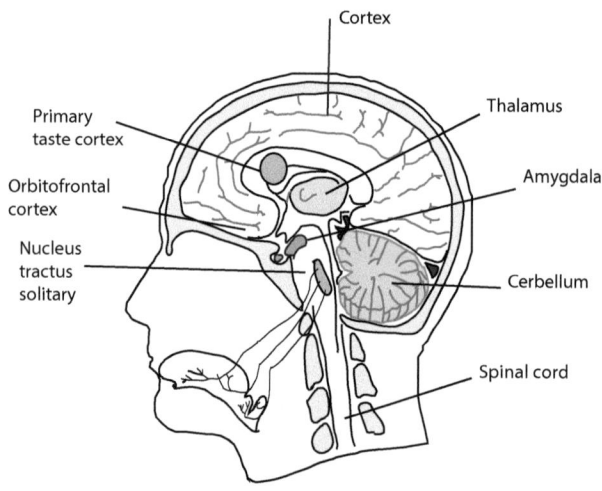

Fig. 2.11 Anatomy of taste.

In the secondary taste center in orbitofrontal cortex is a more complex treatment of taste experience. In orbitofrontal cortex is an identification of the taste and it is a compilation of the various impressions a subject to hazard, palatability, heating/cooling and identification memory, which together give a conscious taste sensation that provides saliva suspension or when food is unfit for use can trigger an automatic vomiting reflex. Even the perception of the body's internal status through hormone, blood glucose level and the feeling of hunger is involved in the orbitofrontal cortex integrated taste experience on the palatability.

Treatment of taste signals is done in a similar way as for the other perception which structurally brings together signals from neurons with the same function or location in the body. Different parts of the tongue are represented together and receptors for sweet are grouped together. This means that when taste receptors are sensitive to several basic flavors get primary taste center nerve signals with complex patterns, which often give the complex flavors such as sweet-sour or bitter-sweet. Sharp flavors that chili pepper gives a hot feeling via temperature receptors, while mint has a cooling sensation via receptors for cooling. The intense equity/assets ratio of a taste sensation is encoded in taste receptors by an increased frequency of action potentials are done through taste nerves to the primary taste center (Insula).

The development of the human sense of taste has been designed in order to ensure good nutrition and avoid unfit for human consumption. Here are some examples of properties of different taste sensations:

• Sweet: Give valuable calorie.

• Salt: supports fluid balance in the body.

• Umami: Protein rich food.

• Acid: Tainting, bad or dangerous food.

• Bitter: poisonous food.

As for the smell, to measure the sensitivity when it comes to taste a distinction is made between the detection threshold for taste where you feel a slight taste difference but to be able to identify the substance while the identification threshold applies for identification of taste. In table 2.2 is given a few concentrations of flavors for to reach the detection threshold. You can see major differences between e.g. sweet tastes where saccharin is up to 400 times sweeter than sucrose. Even sensitivity to bitter taste is big.

Bitter	Quinine sulfate	0,008 µmol/l
Acid	Citic acid	2,3 µmol/l
Sweet	Sackaros	10 µmol/l
	Glucose	80 µmol/l
	Saccharin	0,023 µmol/l
Salt	Sodium chloride	10 µmol/l

Table 2.2   Identification threshold taste

At University in Bristol has English researchers discovered connection between taste sensation and depression (see reference 2.4). Patients who suffer from depression have low levels of serotonin or norepinephrine which gives blunt of taste. The researchers tested healthy volunteers through to give anti-depressants drugs that affect serotonin or norepinephrine levels in the body, to see if these neurotransmitters affect taste experience.

First, the subjects were tested with four topics with sweet, salt, bitter and sour flavor and then got the subjects the antidepressant drugs that increase serotonin or noradrenaline levels in the body. The test was carried out during three different conditions with SSRI drugs which increase serotonin level, shared NARI preparations affecting noradrenalin level and finally the placebo. After two hours was test repeated. The results showed that when serotonin level went up could the subjects feel sweet taste at a much weaker concentration than before. The effect of bitter taste was more dramatic in which people could identify the taste with less than half the concentration than before. For norepinephrine levels was instead an increased sensitivity to bitter and sour taste at lower levels. Taste for salt was not affected at all and the placebo had no effect on taste experience.

The researchers could also note that the subjects who were nervous in ahead of the tests had a more negative impact on levels of taste in bitter and salt. This suggests that a person's mood (feeling) also has an impact on taste. As a result of the research think it that tests of taste in conjunction with depressive condition can help with choosing the right antidepressant drugs. Earlier have physicists given the right antidepressant drugs to patients only in 60-80 % of cases, which often takes up to 4 weeks to identify. Through taste test in conjunction with depression believe they can improve the selection of the right antidepressant.

In the case of other animal species, it has been seen that in some mammals have the receptors for sweet taste mutated so that they are not active. Animals that live on meat have no need of the sweet treat as for example some hyena species and even domestic cats have no taste buds too sweet. Pet owners have found that domestic cats are not especially interested in sweets which on the other hand, dogs are. As humans we are marked by past experience of food. If we become sick of any previous dish we avoid eating the remains. Animal studies have shown the same effect where poisoned food that provided results in vomiting to the animal in the future quite avoid such food with the same taste sensation. At try where you give an audio tone in connection with the prepared food has not received the same effect relating to the aversion to the sound. Scientists believe that the association between sick and taste/smell plays a major role in the survival of the animals.

Synesthesia

As we have seen in the description of human minds are the links between certain perceptions relating to collaborative senses. For the sense of sight for example there were links to the cores of cortex for both audio and tactile information which could control eye movement in the direction where the perception occurred. In the same way are taste sensations linked both to the olfactory and sensory perception via the orbitofrontal cortex.

One other more unusual type of interconnection of mind occurs in persons who have a cognitive ability that is called synesthesia. Generally, synesthesia may arise by interaction between all the five senses but also associations of words and different concepts can occur. Researchers on the topic indicates that it is possible to define 60-150 different types of cognitive connections such as letters have different color, music can give color experiences, first name may provide taste sensations, words can give fragrance experiences, some objects with specific color and shape can provide pain impulses and more common in people with synesthesia is that units of the week day names and month names develops different color experiences. As a person with synesthesia said "I remember people's name days because I feel that the days and months have different color experiences". Synesthesia is experienced as an automatic feature where the most frequently occurring color experiences of letters, numbers or whole words. The opposite of a color gives perception of a letter or number is extremely rare. There are also questions about synesthesia if the ability are depending of color letters that occurs via common sights or occur to certain colors in more associative cortical areas

Synesthesia is a relatively unusual cognitive ability and different researchers provides that ability is of one of 200 peoples, while others specify numbers one of 20000 people, of which 60-70 % are women's. Most common is the ability to see color in conjunction with letters or numbers which are referred to as grapheme type of synesthesia. Corresponding phenomenon with regard to color experience of sound is called the phoneme type synesthesia. Other involved characteristics of synesthesia persons are that they more often are left-handed, certain heredity via X-chromosomes, normal neurologically developed and in many cases, artistic excellence. As examples can be mentioned some famous people: Franz Liszt (composer), Vasilij Kandinsky (painter), Duke Ellington (Orchestra leader), Marilyn Monroe (movie star) and Lady Gaga (singer). Synesthesia ability is characterized by intuition, lasting, constant color experience, can cause emotional experience and affect memory. Many people with synesthesia ability are not aware that these faculties are unusual but have from childhood accepted his ability as completely natural. Often these people are aware of this ability in synesthesia first in adult age.

One can see that the entire chain of perception, and memory affect a person with synesthesia on a deeper level subconsciously. When it comes to for example to remember a person's name will be added to a color experience that is associated with the name and appeared to be easier to create a lasting memory when multiple minds are linked to in this case name (for example, the name Karl associated with color blue). There are two concepts with regard to synesthesia. One specific characteristic are referred to as properties where it is form letters or music sounds which directly determines the experience. In the second case, which is called concept synesthesia, see cognitive functions and learning with which concepts that provide color performance. Research on synesthesia have in recent times been a renaissance when the new imaging techniques, fMRI, MEG , and opportunities to using magnetic stimulation (TMS, TDC'S) control the synapse function in the cortex. This brought about new opportunities to see the brain's work during induced test cases. As we noted in the previous chapter that scientists today are not quite able to explain human consciousness, so has research even for synesthesia ability different theories.

Researcher in psychology, Dr. Devin Terhune at the University of Oxford as a special interest in the field of synesthesia indicates that 85% of his subjects have link between color and other sensory input. These people often have a greater capacity to be able to distinguish between different colors like the previously described persons who have four types of cones in the eye (tetra chromatic).

Terhune describe in a report Current Biology 2011 (see ref. 2.5) for results from experiments with 6 subjects with synesthesia ability with color grapheme in comparison with 6 people with ordinary perception without synesthesia. Intension of the study was to investigate if people with synesthesia are especially sensitive in primary visual cortex (V1) and see what role it plays in synesthesia ability. Attempts were made with two different methods on the one hand, Transcranial Magnetic Stimulation (TMS) and partly with Transcranial Direct Current Stimulation (TDCS). TMS was used for to determine the excitability threshold in primary visual cortex V1 for that person would be able to perceive light flashes in the field of view (darkened laboratory). The test is carried out through to a magnetic coil is held close in this case visual cortex V1 and magnetic pulses generated targeted at selected centers. The results showed that people with synesthesia was 3 times more sensitive to magnetic field (TMS) than people without synesthesia. A comparison was made where TMS pulses were directed against motor cortex and the limit value for to get a muscle in a finger to move itself was measured. In this case was seen no difference between the groups. The study showed that the visual area of cortex V1 has much higher sensibility of those with synesthesia than for those in the control group.

The other method was to use the TDCS for to see if the ability to synesthesia can be modeled by influence of the neural synapses in the primary visual cortex V1. The method affects the neurons threshold for activation so that when the electrode placed at the visual cortex is the cathode reduces the stimulation of neurons and when it is anode is given increased stimulation of neurons. A third item was to give a placebo treatment without power as control function. Subjects performed while tests with different number-color combinations and a Stroop test, then was valued. The experiment showed that the ability to synesthesia was affected to increase or decrease in the pace of that view was enabled cortex V1 by TDCS as anode and cathode. This research indicates that a higher neural sensitivity in primary visual cortex V1 has effect on ability to synesthesia.

Another scholar who has interest in synesthesia is Dr. David Brang at the University of California, which studied various aspects of heredity, neural networks, and more concerning color grapheme type of synesthesia. Brang notes that people with synesthesia ability often have more connections and more gray matter between the sensory areas in which synesthesia associations occur. Researcher can now map the neuron axons (white matter) with the technology "Diffusion Tensor Imaging" (DTI) that shows neuron links via the neural network. Researcher Brang has given out a number of research papers on synesthesia research. In a report from the 2010 published in Neuroimage 53 (see ref. 2.6) described a study in which it examined if it is any link between visual cortex V4 which is involved in color detection and the temporal area of the grapheme, Posterior Temporal Grapheme Area (PTGA). In order to be able to get an idea of how the synesthesia of color occurs used the technique of high resolution MEG, where via the measurement of the brain's own magnetic field can get accurate time resolution of the interesting neuron signals. The study was designed to determine which of two theories about synesthesia as applicable <. One theory claims that synesthesia occurs in a direct link between the two brain areas V1 and PTGA, while the other theory claims that the feedback links in sight path that would normally be cancelled are involved. The measurements showed no difference between the 4 people with synesthesia and the 4 control individuals without synesthesia ability when the activation of area PTGA in the area of grapheme identification. In the visual cortex V4 area was measured, however, a significant difference in activation between the groups. This activation was almost directly (5 ms.) after activation in PTGA. The results of the study showed that the theory of direct link between visual cortex V4 and PTGA area of the grapheme is the likely for people with synesthesia. The researchers summarize the result to be the first group to demonstrate the simultaneous process of color grapheme synesthesia in V4 and PTGA. This proves the theory of direct links between the associated areas in synesthesia. The researchers also note that the next step in the research should investigate the people with synesthesia who get color experience even at the thinking of letters or numbers. Even synesthesia with other combinations of the senses requires further research.

In conclusion, can we say that research on synesthesia have several different theories regarding how the phenomenon occur.

• Synesthesia occurs through more relations between the involved areas of mind and more gray matter.

• Theories on to a synesthesia person's brain think that it would be more like a child's brain before birth where these lines are not completing developmental.

• New links are created between the areas in the brain that normal are separated.

• Synesthesia has a hereditary component dependency of X chromosome and majority is women.

It can be mentioned some cases of synesthesia has yielded very unusual skills. Memory artist Daniel Tammert who has synesthesia ability has been shown to be able to give an account of 22514 decimal digits for the number PI. More interesting case of synesthesia has been investigated by Professor Megan Steven at Dartmouth College in England. In this case were the subject blind sins10 years on the basis of the degeneration of the eye's retina. The person had had normal color sight before blindness. The person John Fullwood has synesthesia experience if you verbally mentions days of the week or months. Days of the week are seen along an oval line with the current and the following week's days with distinct colors for each day of the week. Study by fMRI equipment showing activity in the visual cortex V1 and V4 when you mention for example a day of the week. This shows that the same areas that deal with normal vision and colors experience is enabled when words of the days in a week are treated in the auditory centers of the cortex.

Savant syndrome

In connection with this chapter, heading super senses, the exceptional memory skills and artistic abilities should be mentioned as presented by persons with so called Savant syndrome. Despite that these people suffer from various serious developmental disorders relating to autism and difficulties to cope with normal lives can these people develop exceptional genius talents. Back in the late 1800's described patients with then called "Idiot Savant" by the English physician John Langon Down which, among other things is known for the discovery of the disease Down's syndrome. He described, among other things patients who could quote a book already after just reading the book once and a twelve-year old boy who could multiply three digit numbers faster than they could be written on the paper. With regard to the presence of Savants, research has shown that about 1 out of 1000 mentally retarded is Savant, of which about 10% have autism; they have often IQ lower than 70 and about 6 times more men than women are Savants. From Savants has approximately 50 – 100 people in the world of exceptional skills and called "miracle Savants". Despite their disability presents these people excellent abilities in music, art, mathematics, calendar calculations and super memory. A famous so called miracle Savant is the departed American Kim Peek. He became world famous through that been an idols to the movie "Rain Man" which writes by Barry Morrow as, among other things had contact with Kim during the script work. The actor Dustin Hoffman got an Oscar for best actor and thanked Kim in his acceptance speech for all support during role portrayal. Kim Peek had an unusually large brain but MRI studies showed that he lacked the Corpus Callosum between left and right brain and the cerebellum was malformed. Kim had difficulties with everyday chores and learned first to go at 4 years of age. Early started Kim to read and memorize the books and at the age of six had Kim already memorized the first 8 volumes of the family's encyclopedia by heart. In later life indicates diverse sources that Kim could tell 7600-9000 books by heart, and among these books included the Bible and Shakespeare's complete works. Kim had an ability to directly transfer memories from short-term memory to long-term memory and could read two pages of a book at the same time, with each eye on each book page. Like many people with Savant Syndrome was on the other hand, the ability to understand the proverbs, metaphors and abstract concepts underdeveloped. In addition to this was Kim a big "Crunchers" that could United States all post numbers, geographical facts, historical facts and could instantly figure out what day of the week a certain date had.

Other famous miracle Savants is, among other things. Daniel Tammet an Englishman with the unique ability to multiply large numbers with lightning speed, specify if a big number is a prime number and 2004 at a charity event put Europe record in to read up 22514 decimal places of PI' from the memory. Tammet has appeared in two books "Embracing the wide sky" and the memoirs "Born on a Blue Day". Tammet who is an autistic Savant can fairly accurately describe how he perceives the perception in conjunction with calendar calculations, which otherwise Savants often have difficult to express. Tammet describes how he is experiencing abstract information such as digits in a visually dynamic way. He experiences digits and words with a touch of synesthesia so that they have different former, colors and textures etc. This gives a deeper dimension and help to remember long sequences that e.g. 22514 decimal places of PI. At operations summary or to determine if a number is prime Tammet is experiencing such that the digits form complex multi-dimensional pattern and quick as lightning gives the answers. Even when it comes to language, he sees the cluster in a mental architecture where each vocabulary has a special place for each language. Tammet can speak 8 different languages of which he learned Icelandic in 7 days.

Identical twins George and Charles, Savants described by the neurologist Oliver Sack in the book "the man who confused his wife with a hat". Despite that they barely could put together 2 and 2 could they in lightning speed indicate the exact day of the week for any date in the 80000 years. They were also able to quite exactly specify e.g. the number of matches which was poured out of a box on the floor by a quick glance. Also, computation of long digit primes was carried out quickly. Even in art, for example the English miracle Savant Stephen Wiltshine who has shown an ability to memorize, and then be able to draw detailed pictures of architecture from cities. In conjunction with a television program was Stephen make a short helicopter ride over London and Tokyo and could then take out incredibly detailed images of these cities from memory.

Research regarding brain function of Savants can provide better understanding of the brain's internal work with emphasis on the left and right brain hemisphere different function. A theory on the Savant ability to remember details argue that the normal ability to filter out details from the incoming sent does not work without all the details are saved. Possibly can the non-declarative memory (procedural memory), which is typically used for the learning of procedures that cycling, at Savant use for automat-

94

ic storage of memory impressions. The capacity of Savants, for example quickly figure out which day of the week a certain date have, seems to be instinctively without thinking and in a similar way to the unconscious art of cycling through procedural memory. Some researchers at the University of Oklahoma tested the ability of a normal person to learn methods for calendar calculation. The method was included a 9 pages long table by heart. The subject Benj Langdon practiced a long time and was pretty good at calculating the day of the week but was nowhere near as fast as the previously described the twins George and Charles. But after a while, he discovered that the speed increased dramatically. His brain had made a breakthrough and was able to do calculations without to consciously go through calculation steps one by one. Scientists believe that the calculations programmed into the right brain and thereby become parallel, unconscious and fast.

A recurring phenomenon of Savants is to the left hemisphere has congenital deformities or have been injured in any accident. In the majority of 90 % of the population are left hemisphere dominant when it comes to abstract thinking and consciousness. The left hemisphere tinning lobe is therefore part of the filter that sorts sent and select out the relevant information. This and brain plasticity is probably behind that persons with Savant syndrome to a greater extent use the right detailed focused brain. This relationship is strengthened by the fact that healthy persons that by an accident received injuries in the left tinning lobe suddenly can get Savant ability in new previously not use areas of knowledge. Some researchers believe that the preponderance of male Savants can depend on congenital birth defects in the left hemisphere. This would depend on that fetus exposed to high testosterone halter during pregnancy which left hemisphere is more delicate for when it developed more slowly. When it comes to acquired Savant syndrome from an injury can the history of Orlando Serell a 10 year old boy in connection with the baseball games got the ball with force in the left tinning lobe and was knocked to the ground. He was able to get up after a while and play on. Orlando felt that he had a new ability that in detail to remember everything. If you mentioned a specific date, he was able to say which day of the week that was, what happened on this day and the weather had been. This shows that Savant ability usually associated with lesions in the left tinning lobe and can occur spontaneously in connection with an injury.

A researcher who has taken up this issue is Professor Allan Snyder at the University of Sydney in Australia. Snyder set the hypothetical question of whether one can exercise up Savant skills with ordinary people by to disturb out left hemisphere tinning lobe. By try cancel the left brain hemisphere tinning lobe by means of repetitive Transcranial Magnetic Stimulation (rTMS) tested if subject's Savant skills can be developed. By that point a coil near the temporal lobe on the left side of the head and repetitive send magnetic pulses with rTMS equipment can the brain be provisionally inhibit in this area. In one of the trials were 4 of 11 participants a more detailed ways to draw after stimulation. Even induce to flawless proofreading was improved. Checks for any hour showed that ability remained short-lived. Snyder argues that attempts to support the hypothesis that it can activate Savant skills in the right hemisphere by using rTMS technology by suppress left tinning lobe and thereby reduce the usual filtering of perception in the left side of the brain. These attempts are in an early stage where the technology for rTMS needs to be refined in order to more precisely control the inhibitory magnetic fields.

Professor Snyder is also involved in trials with Transcranial Direct Current Stimulation, TDCS in order to see if it can affect creativity when it comes to solving problems where some sort of new insight is required. The problems were designed as a logical mathematic expression where an equal sign in the middle would show two equivalent expressions. Digits were Roman numbers laid out with matches and in the task you would move a match for that expression would be correct. The task required need to think "outside the box" in order to find the correct solution. The experiment was carried out in three different conditions: a placebo treatment where no current TDCS was given, on the one hand, a treatment in which the left head tinning lobe cathode connected and right tinning lobe had anode attached and finally there was the anode is connected to the left tinning lobe and cathode to the right tinning lob. Intension with TDCS treatment is that the side with the cathode connected inhibits neurons activity potential and with the anode stimulates activity potential. The attempt by taken with 60 healthy subjects at the University of Sydney (see ref. 2.7). Activation was with the DC 1.6 mA for 10 minutes with a stepping up and down traps during 30 seconds. At comparison of settlement rate for the more difficult problem could just 20 % of the subjects to solve it when placebo treatment lasted while 60% managed to solve the problem in dealing with the cathode on the left side and anode on the right side of the parietal lobe. The other case gave the same effect as placebo. We also saw that people more quickly found the solution to the task. Professor Snyder believes that this attempt demonstrates the hypothesis that left tinning lobe have an effect which can inhibit new insights in creative This probably then a filtering vis-à-vis earlier saved methods can inhibit innovation. While the right tinning lobe is associated with innovative thinking and identification of new not previously identified pattern. The researchers suggest more attempts for that clarify the mechanisms behind these effects.

In the animal world there are the more "super senses" which provides extended ability to orient themselves and feel of booty animals. Homing pigeons have for example ability to sense the Earth's magnetic field which through their nervous system helps to navigate home to nest even far away from. The Arctic tern which flies 2,000 miles between the Arctic and Antarctica are navigating with the help of the polarized light from the Sun which created from particles in the atmosphere. Animals such as mice, cats and seals have very sensitive whiskers where for example a mouse can sense even the slightest air current. Sharks have electric sensory cells in the nose that can detect small impulses from muscle movement of fishermen swap. A way for people to get "super senses" is with the help of various technical innovations. We may, for example see in almost total darkness with special infrared glasses used in military contexts. When it comes to the whales which singing in the inaudible range below 10 Hz, can be heard with microphone and amplifier transform sound into the audible range for us human. Even the dolphin's ultrasound vocalizations can similarly be transposed to the audible range.

This chapter has a mapping of the different senses to show on the limits of our perception. The large amount of information, about 11 Mbit/sec, which is constantly bombardment our brain cannot be handled in the consciousness. Why is parallel processing of the various signals of the senses in different parts of cortex and compiled to about 40 bit/second that our consciousness can manage. Evolution has created automatic unconscious processing of dangerous situations by, among other things amygdala treatment of incoming signals, which evaluates a potential threat and in some cases enable the body's defense mechanisms. In the following chapters will be shown on how we are affected by body language, intuition and unconscious perception acts in the "The Unconscious Zone".

Chapter 7 Can brain be hacked?

Introduction

Chapter 3 Can brain be hacked?

Mindreading

In this chapter asks if you can create equipment in order to be able read thoughts, control the behavior or directly transfer information between connected brains. When you examine the current research are the many results pointing in this direction. The remainder of this article describes a number of research projects in which the man with the new methods have been able to identify the brain's way of working and by computers even been able to identify pattern in thoughts.

In the extension of these results, there are different ways to be able to affect a brain on an unconscious level, among other things with the help of the sense of smell, investigate criminals with advanced lie detectors or able to investigate inside dreams. The different senses such as vision, hearing and tactile features identify the areas of the cortex where the primary input is received (see fig. 2.2). Mapping has also been about where the respective neurons for individual nerve signals are represented. Maps view (retina topic), hearing (tone topic) and sensory (somatic topic) has been developed. This information can be used for analysis of fMRI signals where a selection of interesting brain areas can be studied.

Image interpretation through Visual cortex

There is an intense research on the possibilities to detect how the brain handles images in visual cortex. It makes use of fMRI methods for identification of the involved areas of the cortex. One of the reasons for this research is that the visual perception probably reflects the brain's general approach. As we have seen in Chapter 2 is the brain's visual processing complex with processing of input in many different support centers (V1 ... V8). With the help of fMRI, it is possible to get a detailed picture of the brain's activity with good spatial resolution. It terms the smallest parts in these fMRI images to voxel and they have a resolution down to about 1x1x1 mm. In early experiments with fMRI technology was used simple images as crosses, triangles or lines to identify which areas of the visual cortex that are activated in image interpretation. These attempts were relatively limited as man in a less amount of images was able to identify the image as the subject viewed. In these cases had been previously stored fMRI-information about all images for comparison.

Professor Jack Gallant that works at the University of California Berkeley has later carried out a number of studies in order to identify how the brain processes the sights. One of the ideas behind the study was to investigate if it is possible to build up a library of pattern recognition of visual images that can be interpreted by a computer algorithm. The method is based on observing all visual areas in the cortex simultaneously with fMRI and through catalogs of computer algorithms to process the image entire complex patterns (multivariate pattern analysis, MVPA).

Gallant has in an article in Neuron (ref. 3.1), reported on a research project with fMRI examined three subjects who consider a number of black/white photos. It looked especially three areas in the visual cortex (V1, V2, V3), (V3A, V3B, V4, LO) and anterior occipital cortex (AOC), see figure 2.4. The experiment was set up so that people first see 1750 different black/white photographs where fMRI images were stored for each photograph. Then appeared 120 all new photographs in which new fMRI images stored, after which an analysis was made with various computer algorithms to be able to recreate the photograph and classify the content of the 120 photographs.

The aim of the research was to develop a self-learning computer algorithm that can classify a common photography outbound from its various parameters. Common photographs have a complex statistical structure and a rich semantic content. This task is far more advanced than that in the previous attempt to identify known patterns in an image. In order to be able to create a probability model in which each voxel in the image coded of a computer algorithm used fMRI data from the 1750 testing images as a database for coding of the computer model's parameters. Analysis of image content involves two stages where the first coded structural data from the early visual areas (V1, V2, and V3). Thereafter codes the semantic content from the higher visual areas. In the model for pairing of semantic variables there are defined 23 different semantic properties for an image. The semantic categories are selected specifically to provide unambiguous classified rules. Examples of the selected categories are: crowd, portrait, people, water, land, birds ... indoors, outdoors etc. The semantic model provides three outputs on the treated photo: similar to category, similar to no category or have no importance. In likelihood algorithm is then made a complete treatment of all data which result in a probability calculation for current slide that can be compared against previous images in the database. The combination of structural data and semantic data in this computer model gives a much better result than previous use models. The researchers also did reconstruction attempt of the 120 images, where the comparison was made against an image database of 6 million images from internet. One can of course not recreate exact copies of the original image from fMRI data, but the results showed great conformity with the structural and semantic content of the selected images.

The research group around Jack Gallant has taken another step which made algorithms in order to be able to encoding with and reconstruct the video films. In a report in Current Biology, 21 2011 (see ref. 3.2) shows a method to filter mobile information from fMRI signals when a subject looks at short videos. The model is built around the analysis of fMRI data in the primary visual areas V1, V2 and V3. Attempts were undertaken with three volunteers who got to see video clips downloaded from You Tube on the internet. In this case, it was managed individual adaptation of algorithms for each trial subject. For the collection of test data to the computer model were performed fMRI scans of the subjects in 12 pass with 10 minutes of video viewing at a time. Walks of life contained 10-20 second sequences randomly selected and each video were shown one time. These fMRI data was used to build up the computer model for coding of algorithm parameters. In these algorithms performed a number of filtrations for to catch the energy in movements and the dynamic blood flow in each voxel.

The results from these trials have shown that it is surprisingly good, can show much of a movie's momentum from fMRI data. When the subjects have been see new cut scenes that repeated 9 times with 10 minutes each time, so have you been able to rebuild cut scenes out of recorded fMRI data. For example, in a video clip that was evaluated was shown an elephant walking in a desert landscape and the reconstruction gave a Dumbo like formation wandering across the screen. The reconstructed video sequence with current technology just show general movement, form and color for objects but has no finer detail and facial expression. Gallant sees a potential to with new input from equipment with e.g. better resolution in fMRI images to improve the level of detail in the reconstruction of the video sequence.

These research results are only useful for research on-going how the brain's visual cortex works and mapping of the visual perception by direct visual information through the eyes. The use of these research findings can affect many neurological medical conditions where it is possible to identify, for example visible problem, cognitive disease, stroke or hallucination. Another aspect of this research is that some of these areas in the visual cortex is also involved in the dreams and relive visual memories. Even in these areas, there is a wide research.

There is research on the visual cortex in in conjunction with dreams going on in Japan at the ATR Computational Neuroscience in Kyoto. Scientists Yukiyasu Kamitani has conducted a study in which he investigated three subjects with fMRI and EEG registrations of visual cortex during sleep. When using EEG registrations discovered the dream state in the early sleep phase the person has been waked and shall provide a report on the dream content. Total has each person registered about 200 times over a number of days. The researchers identified the 20 most common objects that entered in dream descriptions.

In order to be able to identify the content of dreams in fMRI images made registrations with fMRI where a number of videos with relevant content were displayed. These inputs were fed into a computer algorithm for parameter setting of a decoder for each test subject. The results showed that the man through the analysis of fMRI data from approximately 10 seconds before awakening could enter simple connection like a car, a person etc. with 75-80% certainty.

Research shows that the higher cortical areas in the visual cortex have similar representation in dreams as in visual information through the eyes. These points on that even visual fantasy are represented in these areas. It also points out that the dreams in these cases generated in short-term memory when compliance with the analysis results can be found in max ca10 seconds before awakening. The researchers are aiming to further studies investigate fMRI registrations during REM sleep which require longer trial time when REM sleep normally requires a minimum of 45 minutes of sleep.

Decoding of hippocampus and prefrontal lobe

Another area of research with fMRI is a study of the brain's hippocampus area on memory storage of location information. The Nobel Prize in medicine in 2014 was divided between the researchers John O'Keefe due from England and spouses Moser from Norway for the discovery of "place cells" in the hippocampus. The Nobel laureates have discovered a positioning system, an "internal GPS" in the brain that make it possible to orient themselves in the room. When a rat be found himself at a specific location in a room always was activated certain nerve cells in the part of the brain that is called the hippocampus. Other neurons in the hippocampus were activated at other locations in the room. O'Keefe drew the conclusion that these "place cells" in the brain form a kind of internal map of the room. The hippocampus is involved in several tasks like to navigate in our surroundings, store and recall memories and by perceptions of future events.

A team of scientists under the leadership of Demis Hassabis at University College London has examined subjects with fMRI as tested in a virtual spatial environment (see ref. 3.4). Computing environment is shaped by one blue and one green room, with four distinct observation points in each room. Some simple objects as a door, chair, plate and a watch were in each room for to facilitate orientation. The test was made in two stages where the first fMRI data were collected during subject's hiking in rooms with stops at the 8 observation points. These fMRI data was used to control parameters in an algorithm for analysis of fMRI data. The results showed that could then predict the observation point the subject is in front off. In the computer model gives fMRI data from the hippocampus area data for observational site while data from the hippocampal gyrus pointing out in which room (blue or green) person is. This type of information would in the future be able to show whether a suspected person for a particular crime have result from the crime scene.

Research on decision-making in the prefrontal lobes has been tested under the leadership of Professor John-Dylan Haynes at the Max Planck institutes in Leipzig. A study of 3 male and 5 female students were made to determine if via fMRI can register the intentions (selection) between different options from the medial prefrontal lobes (see ref. 3.5). The experiment was carried out by volunteers were instructed to take a decision to either subtract or add two numbers after a command word on the screen. After a waiting period of between 2.7 to 10.8 seconds was the object presented two numbers on the monitor as the person performing the selected operation with. After further 2 seconds appeared 4 numbers on screen, of which 2 were correct numbers for addition and subtraction. The other two numbers was inaccurate random numbers. The subject chose the number that corresponded to the rendered operation by pressing the 4 different keys. There first were made a number of attempts to find the appropriate parameters to the computer model's algorithm. Then test to carry out experiments to with the help of the computer model predict the outcome in a number of new trials. The results showed that 75% of the attempts could predict the outcome which is significantly better than chance. The researchers believe that it is a first step in to be able to identify thoughts from fMRI data. The next step in the research is to see if you can recognize the intention in fMRI data already before a person becomes conscious of its decision (subconsciously).

Another interesting research using fMRI have been carried out by researcher Adrian Owen when at the University of Cambridge, UK. Owen tested back in 1997, a 26 year old female patient who through a virus infection of the brain ended up in a coma. The female patient was after that virus infection healed out left in a vegetative state. These patients in vegetative state has often come out of a state of coma which ended up in a state where the show vague emotions but not any awareness about environment. Owen had earlier in healthy subjects experience of an area of the brain known as the fusiform face area (FFA) is activated when you see a familiar face. Owen patient tested with fMRI and could see that the (FFA) area was activated strongly when the patient saw the photo on a familiar face. The female patient was found to have left significantly brain function and was able to return after rehabilitation have an active life, but then in a wheelchair. This patient could later write a book about the experiences and could express the frustration she felt during the time she was assumed to be unconscious during the diagnosis of vegetative state.

Owen published 2006 an article in Science 313 on a 23 year old woman who ended up in a vegetative state at a car accident. In this case, was chosen a different approach where the patient gave two different responses for answer choices yes or no. She was asked to imagine her selves playing tennis for the option yes, which in healthy people enable "supplementary motor cortex" in the brain. While she is in no option would think of wandering around in his home, which in healthy people enables hippocampal gyrus in the inner part of the brain. The patient who had been in vegetative state in 5 months after the accident showed a similar response in the brain as healthy people when relevant yes or no questions were put to her. The article attracted huge attention where two opinions emerged. On the other hand, felt some neurologists that the phenomenon was descended from unconscious reactions in the brain, while others saw a future potential for rehabilitation of these painter. See Ref. 3.6 for a comprehensive report on this research in respect of vegetative state.

Owen got the offer to start a further development of the method at the University of Western Ontario in Canada. He has continued development of measurement methods with test of a portable EEG equipment to be able to treat patients in their home environment. This equipment is much cheaper and can detect that a yes is represented by a hand/finger movement while a no through movement of the toes. This research may lead to a revolution in the treatment and rehabilitation of patients in vegetative State.

Method electrocorteography (ECoG)

It is carried out also research with methods that operate in electrodes directly into the brain. A method that is called electrocorteography (ECoG) means to operate in a matrix of electrodes in the skull on the surface of the cerebral cortex. This research is carried out, among other things on the New York State Department of health's Wadesworth Centre in Albany by researcher Gerwin Schalk. Because you comes under the bones and skin to you get much better signal quality from neurons electrical activity. Research is done in the context of surgical treatment of patients with severe epileptic seizures where the skull is opened for localization and removal of tissue involved in the assault. Through to connect the implanted electrode matrix to computer equipment can a detail record of the signal patterns that occur at different thoughts. Through evaluation by learning software witch can identify patterns in EEG signals that could be used for e.g. control of a denture. Schalk shows in a video how a patient can maneuver a virtual hand on a monitor by just thinking about moving their hands. The method could be useful for example for patients who are paralyzing due spine cord damage (see ref. 3.7).

The method is useful for detection of nerve signals in a large number of centers in the brain. The scientists has in a study investigating how the brain generates speech then you either speak high or when you repeat a word for yourself. A surprising discovery is a great difference between the high speaking and thinking of words. At normal speech-generating brain generate two signals. One signal manages how the muscles and oral cavity to move itself. While the other signal activate the brain's auditory cortex. When the person only thinks of a word is generated no muscle tone but enable the auditory cortex. You can like this to listen to your own supposed speech. This can be a way in a future to record a person's thinking. This method of directly into the brain to be able to reach different centers in the cortex can give very detailed knowledge about the mechanisms of the brain's control.

A different example of the ECoG research in Albany has been carried out under the direction of Peter Brunner (see ref. 3.8). Seven patients were scanned through EEG equipment when they read aloud from a number of different texts in order to store a library of brain activity in the auditory cortex (mostly in the temporal lobe). By signal processing of gamma activity in brain waves could create models for the use of phonemes and with learning algorithms create a library. When the subjects then quietly thought of the corresponding sentences it was possible in a computer program to recreate these sentences via EEG signal and printing them on a printer. Today, this requires that the electrodes are posted at cortex surface under the skull. But in the future maybe we can use external electrodes for EEG recording. This would be able to be an opportunity for an ALS patient to directly communicate with the environment.

Synthetic telepathy via EEG signals

Try to use "synthetic telepathy " by EEG signals going on at the University of California under the direction of professor Mike D due Zumra. Research carried out with funds from the US Army for use in silent communication on the battlefield but can also have uses for stroke patients or other neurological diseases. Research areas include automatic speech recognition fMRI imaging and Brain-computer interface via EEG signals. The goal is to integrate 128 EEG electrodes in a protective helmet for use in battlefield. The research concerns the possibility that by EEG pattern recognition of the internal monologue at the supposed speech and self-learning algorithms to identify a person's thoughts. It includes the equipment need to be calibrated for each carrier. The next step is to via electrical signals (radio or internet) to transmit these messages to one or multiple target peoples. The target person shall be able to detect e.g. a sentence phrase via an earphone from a synthetic voice. Tests in the investigation has shown that it is possible to transfer Morse coded information via two different supposed expression as a symbol for fluent with Morse code 1 or 0. Final results from this research have yet been published.

A similar research project under the guidance of Professor Rajesh Rao with synthetic telepathy has been carried out at the University of Washington (see ref. 3.12). In this case, have you started from a person who plays a computer game in which a cannon will be fired in the correct moment for to shoot down an attacking missile. This person has a hat with a larger number of electrodes for recording of EEC signaler. Via a self-learning algorithm evaluates EEG signals from motor area of the cortex in order to recognize the touch of a button with e.g. right index finger. This decoded signal is sent via the Internet to a test subject in a different building. This person can't see computer game screen without sitting in front of a keyboard ready to press on a trigger bottom. By TMS the equipment can you give a magnetic pulse to the corresponding motor area for the right index finger to the test subject. The results showed that the man in this study could see that communication link worked brilliantly and led a firing at the right time. In his summary indicates researchers with EEG/TMS equipment can shape a transfer via data link as "brain -to- brain interface". We also see opportunities for transfer of visual and auditory signals in a future with this "non-invasive" method.

Research on the influence of human emotional system is going on at the MIT Media Lab in the United States. Researcher professor Rosalind Picard has at their institution Affective Computing Research group has taken up a portable computer system for identification of a person's emotional state (see Ref. 3.9). In this case, the research focused on to identify facial expressions and head movements of a person and through a probability algorithm able to read a person's emotional state.

The research is designed to help autistic people with interpretation of body language as these people often have problems with social contacts. The system consists of a mini computer that can be fixed in the wearer's waist strap and is connected to a mini camera. The camera can either be directed towards the own face (self-Cam) or against a different conversing person. Computer algorithms follows 24 points on the face through the detection of movement, form and color of these points and can identify 20 countenance and head movement (for example. the main twist or movement of month). In addition the computer detected eleven different communicative movements such as smiling, eyebrow movement or nod. By a Bayesian network model can you follow the person's emotional status. The system continuously evaluates the probability that a person is in one of the 6 different emotional states. These conditions are: consent, aversion, interest, confused, concentrated and thoughtful. Information can be viewed either as a color coded image sweeps in real time or an acoustic information in one earpiece. This appliance has been assessed in connection with training of acoustic people in social interaction. This type of computer communication can also be used for transmission of emotional information to a controlled humanoid robot.

Brain influence via TDCS and TMS

When it comes to how we can affect the brain, there are today several methods were used to directly affect the synapses in the brain cortex. Large interest appears today on the method to via two electrodes on the scalp send weak direct current (1-2 mA) into brain by TDCS (Transcranial direct current stimulation). As described in Chapter 2 of savants to get an inhibition of neurons action potential at the cathode (-) and the corresponding stimulate at the anode (+). A number of research projects have among other things reported that this can increase learning ability by about 30%.

Researcher Andy McKinley at the Air Force Research Laboratory has for the U.S. air force conducted research on image analysis with the help of TDCS (see ref. 3.10). When you perform drone attacks staff sit in command centers far away from the attacked area. From reconnaissance cameras in the drone can you obtain images for analysis in targets of interest. Often, are these shots noisy and have a resolution that makes it difficult to safely identify for example robot ramps. McKinley has in a mission from air force investigated whether to shorten training time for the staff to make target analysis. Earlier has it taken quite a long time for to be trained in being able to make safe target analysis of these images.

The study was carried out with 27 volunteers from the air force and was divided in in three groups 1 and 2 had relevant stimulation while group 3 received placebo (Sham) treatment. The positive electrode (anode) for TDCS equipment was put on the scalp above the area where visual information interpreted in the cortex (ventral-lateral prefrontal cortex (VLPFC)). In this case the electrode was placed on the right side of the head, because this area is most active during visual image analysis. The negative electrode (cathode) was placed in the back of the neck. This stimulation affects synapses in VLPFC to become more active. The results showed that those who received stimulation via TDCS generated 25 % better results by training and made fewer mistakes. Method with the TDCS has also been used in research on the influence among others in decision making, working memory, implicit learning and visual image analysis.

The Method Transcranial Magnetic Stimulation (TMS) is a different method that directly affects the synapses in the brain. In this case there is used a directed strong magnetic field using a magnetic coil that is held above the area of the cortex to be affected. These pulses can be generated as single or repetitive pulses with different interval rTMS (repetitive TMS). In research uses TMS often for to block any part of the cortex. Dependence of parameters as the magnetic field strength and repetitive frequency is the influence of different strength in the exposed area. As we saw in Chapter 2 about savants can these type of expose simulate a Savant like function in the cortex by the TMS.

At clinical trials it have been demonstrated that TMS treatment can affect certain neurological medical conditions such as depression (see Ref. 3. 11). In Sweden has the psychiatrist Vagn Liest treated more than 300 patients against depression with help of rTMS. The treatment is made at a point over the patient's left prefrontal lobe. During about 10 minutes sent repetitive magnetic pulses out which in total gives about 2000 pulses per treatment. This treatment has taken place when antidepressants have not had the intended effect. Liest indicates that 60% of these patients became good or better by the treatment.

Unconscious influences through the sense of smell

Research on the influence of the brain via the human sense of smell is in progress, among other things at Weizmann Institute of Science, Israel under the leadership of Ilana Hairston. Human olfactory sense of smell is in difference from other perception directly related to the brain's cortex without passing through the thalamus. Thalamus deploys other perception to the parts of the cortex for the sense, for example sight to the visual cortex. When we sleep works the thalamus as a gatekeeper and exclude sent to these areas in to the cortex. On the other hand, the sense of smell enabled even during sleep phase.

In one study has it been shown that via this smell channel can a person be affected unconsciously during sleep. In a test series is the people in sleeping phase first exposed to the olfactory system by a pleasant scent at the same time as a weak high-frequency tone is played. Then, it has exposed the olfactory mind of a foul-smelling odor (putrid fish) at the same time with a low frequency tone. By measuring respiration can register deep breaths at the pleasant scent and restrained breathing in phase with the foul-smelling scent. When the subject wakes and when they played up these two tones that were given during sleep and measured up similar reaction in the respiratory frequency during sleep phase. You can liken this unconscious influence of the brain on Pavlov's experiments with dogs which gives a conditioned reflex. The application of these results can be that via scent/hearing program in new knowledge. A risk may be to program on a person's attitude to for example a politicians/politics through to give the foul smell at the same time that a politician's speech is played up. This can give a conditioned reflex in which the person unconsciousness programmed on to perceive the politician in a repulsive way.

As was mentioned in the introduction of this chapter shows the current reaches on the brain to opportunities in a future able to penetrate deep into a person's intimate realm and subconsciously affect a human. That means many opportunities to help people with various neurological disorders but sets also requirements on that it is ethical rules that preserve a person's with.

In his book "1984" takes the author George Orwell up a vision of the future, dystopia, where a dictatorship with access to advanced surveillance technology can have total control of its citizen. This vision has today with all the technology like cell phones with built-in GPS, apps, Facebook, and London 1000 's of surveillance cameras have already begun to monitor and provide full visibility into a citizen life.

It is already today companies like via algorithms can analyze metadata from internet and predict hot spots, monitor suspicious people's movements and check consumer buying. This development has as most new research results a positive and even a risky site where a future dictatorship can get total mind control over its citizens. It is to be hoped that the technological development is guided up so that these aberrations are minimized.

In this chapter accounted for a number of research projects through the new methods with fMRI, MEG, EEG, TDC and TMS can provide a detailed picture of the brain's internal work. Method of fMRI have provided a greater understanding of the visual areas in the cortex and even brought opportunities to recreate the visual dreams. Analysis of auditory cortex has demonstrated the ability to identify a person's inner monologue. EEG equipment that is relatively cheap, is projected to have a large usage especially for disabled and for communication in case of neurological diseases. Research of method electrocorteography (ECoG), in which arrays of electrodes surgically inserted in the skull at top of the cortex can give much information where computer registration directly, can be signal processing. As a result can provide advanced algorithms for control of prostheses or can provide ALS patient is able to communicate. That conclusion on this future scenario may one hope that this development will be guided by ethical rules in order to preserve the personal integrity.

Chapter 4 Body consciousness

Budo the intuitive art of defensive

The concept of body consciousness affects various aspects of how the body works, in one way with the unconscious automated functions such as breathing, heart rate and thermal and partly with a body consciousness where learned movement patterns can be developed without the participation of the usual slow mind. In different parts of the body can also experience traumatic events have left an imprint in the tense muscle memories.

In addition to the five senses sight, hearing, smell, taste and touch that it is often considered being the minds that the brain uses for incoming perception, so believe many that the balance system and body consciousness is our sixth sense that inform the brain about the body's position in relation to its surroundings. Later in this chapter suggests that this body's sixth sense can play role in how training in budo can activate hidden sensations of danger which can be vulnerable in a danger situation. A simple activity like walking requires very complex patterns in the signals that coordinate muscle activity in all the legs and arm muscles that shall be activated. Popular expression is that some movements "sits in spinal cord", see figure 1.1.

The part of the brain that coordinates and controls the body's fine motor movements called the cerebellum and is located low down in the rear part of the brain and is connected to the brain stem and on to extended spinal cord (see fig. 1.3). Conscious movement controls from a different part of the cerebrum and activate parts of the cerebellum. In the cerebellum are stored fine motor movement memories as you have been training in. At for example cycling so has a child difficult to coordinate balance and muscle movement in order to not fall. When you to train up balance ability it is to stored motion memories in the cerebellum. Witch enable when you once learned to ride a bike so mastered that the rest of your lives. In the same way involves exercise of the body within for example sport and martial arts that operating memories are stored and the body performs these programmed movements intuitively without consciousness need to be connected.

As exemplification of how body consciousness is working in "The Unconscious Zone", this chapter is focused on Budo sport Aikido when own experience of training in Aikido, Tai chi, Qi gong and Yoga brought experience of how this training affects the body consciousness.

To get the full understanding of both the physical and mental activity at the training of budo sport, so begins the description of a brief historical overview of how martial arts plant up from the worrier class in the ancient Japan and the Buddhist Zen culture.

During the later decades of the 20th century has the Western world interest in fighting sports that has spread from Japan and China. In Japan is the under the collective name of budo that was traditionally the art of fencing (Kendo), archery (Kyudo) and ju-jutsu. The word Do, which included several Japanese budo sports, can be translated with the road. Out of the earlier schools of martial arts, it has developed more modern variants of budo which purely techniques in order to standardize budo sport and be in bring the graduation of practitioners and start competitions in some schools. Budo lecturer bound in Sweden today has a number of under groups such as Kendo, Karate, Judo, Aikido and ju-jutsu. The increasing interest in the Western world led to budo sport Judo (the soft way) 1964 was introduced as a discipline in the Olympic Games.

Bushido the Samurai's Code of honor

The origins of budo sports in Japan developed in the Warrior class whose practitioners are referred to as Samurais. Historically from 1000 century onwards has been a feudal Japan society with a large number of headman's who had their own armies for defense of their cargo and which are often low in war with other clans to conquer new ground. Centrally located in the country, there was aristocracy which maintained the Japanese emperor to which headman's gave promises of obedience. During 1200 century serious clashes between the two most powerful Warrior nights Tai-

117

ra and Minamato, in which case Taira dynasty had been destroyed. Director Yoritomo for Minamato dynasty was the country's strongest man and took the title Shogun (equivalent to Chief of staff). He created an administrative system in order to check the various clans and warriors affairs, called Shoguanat, in which the emperor was head.

The Shogun system came to endure to the end of 1900-century and the Shoguns was chosen by tradition in the Minamato dynasty. Shogunate conditions induced to the Shogun could control the entire Japan militarily. By the Japan Emperor's religious functions in the Shinto religion he was held up the appearances that he was the ruler of Japan.

The new system entailed the shogunate induced that the professional Warrior was given a high status and warrior families took the important role in the society. Thus became the Warrior (bushi) profession hereditary and children within the samurai families got early learn Warrior's role through ascetic practice, Spartan virtues and self-discipline. The image of the Samurai as selfless, loyal, physical and mental endurance became a role model for every Japan. Much of modern society in Japan stems from the philosophy of the Samurai class.

Samurai was ruled by a code of honor called Bushido which translated means ' Warrior's way '. Bushido spirit was transmitted by oral tradition within the Samurai class and the kids brought up according to bushido spirit. Much of Bushido spirit lives on in Japan and is behind the country's immense technical and economic progress. Prominent properties according to bushido's ethical rules are courage, perseverance, courtesy, duty, loyalty and honor. Etiquette rules in Bushido are extensive and the worst affront for a Japan is to "lose his face". On the surface, a discourtesy met with an adamant face of a Japan without that disrupts the balance. During the 2nd World War held the Japanese to Americans was uncontrolled barbarians who could react strongly to single words, which Japan would not show to the outside world. It is difficult for a Westerner to come in in the Japanese culture and not violate all the unspoken rituals.

At 500 century in China emerged a branch of Mahayana Buddhism called Zen. From China, Zen spread to nearby countries like Korea, Japan and Vietnam. The word Zen in Japanese is a translation from the Chinese (chàn) that can be interpreted meditation. Despite translation of Zen to meditation denotes no passive way to sit and meditate instead there is a high degree an active way to live. Zen has played a large role in the Japanese culture then 1100's and influenced martial arts sports.

The main principles of the doctrine were to man through extreme physical discipline should seek out front to intuitive insight about things and life. A couple of the great theorists in context can be mentioned: Takuan (1573-1645) abbot of the Daitokuji Zen-temple in Kyoto that , among other things wrote a famous letter about fencing art and on the other hand, the complete Japanese introduction of Zen teachings attributed to the Zen master Hakuin (1685-1768).

Zen training intention is to put the mind in a state of the spontaneous intelligence, which can be found in the human subconscious, may operate freely without consciousness prevents it. Zen's main objective is to put the mind in a State of non-consciousness. This is a case where our reference borders, thoughts and psychological restrictions cease to block our subconscious. It achieves a maximum of consciousness, when the instinctive and intuitive assumes command. Zen man lets his natural prevail but to prevent it through acquired blocking. Zen attaches not either the intellectual understanding different value than to be used for communication between people. A quote from a Zen master illumination the issue: "the minds will always react like a ball in a mountain stream", that thoughts must not get stuck or looping around something that can keep them alive. Thoughts will follow thoughts without hesitation or delay.

These thought processes occupy our full attention and as a result, our intuitive reception of sensory input is blocked. In order to be able to react without loss of time and act in the right way requires that the intuition server. When this can be done is to the human being in a state of full life as Zen puts it.

119

Zen purpose is to make the mind calm, so that all thoughts shall be reflected back from its surface, nothing will be able to get caught up and prevent the natural intelligence. Zen man strives to get in a State where the conscious mind cannot hinder the spontaneous intelligence and was also way of the goal.

Zen Buddhism in Japan has in addition in budo also influenced many Japanese in the everyday life through special learning methods. Practical chores are systematic and developed into different so-called roads (do) and each Zen-do leading up to the goal that enlightened State or satori. The who from the beginning was ordinary housework or almost every craft in Japan can be perceived as a Zen-do, with examples such as arranging flowers, raking the yard, formal calligraphy, tea ceremony or sword manufacturing.

Zen art is a combination of random natural elements and the natural control of the tools to use to make the crop product visible to the eye. Zen is thus a practical philosophy, whose principles cannot be learned, and, of course, they have to be experienced through practice. A large group of these Zen-roads are the practical exercises of combat and struggle to do. The Warrior (bushi) practiced Zen in his special way in the actual exercises he was used to. Bushido spirit bred even the warrior to gentleness by practicing Zen-do where music, letter quality poetry was equal pursuits with exercises in battle.

Warrior's gear was for many centuries various types of swords and the developed schools within the Samurai class where different champion streamline the exercises in how a sword would be handled in the battle for survival. Samurai bar usually a short and a long sword called daisho. A renowned sword master was Miyamoto Musashi (1584-1645) who was famous for having made a large number of duels without any time lost. He founded a school of sword art called "two sky's single school", or two sword school. Musashi wrote 1643 book "Five rings book" (Ref. 4.2), Go rin no sho, about the sword art which is one of Japan's great classic even today.

In parallel with the schools of sword Arts developed schools that was used when the Warrior's own sword broken off and was forced to fight against the armed enemy with the short piece that was left or with just your hands. This fighting style was called Kumiuchi and occurred at 1100's in fighting between Tiara and Minamoto clans. Kumiuchi technology is included also in modern Kendo. These techniques continued to be developed by masters and experts in various areas, which drew up their own techniques and ideas to a special style named Ryu, Ryuha or Ryugi. The first jujutsu school was founded in 1532 and was given the name Takeuchi-ryu and received the largest and fastest expansion. A large number of jujutsu schools was established during the following centuries. Then I myself pursued the modern budo sport Aikido, so will the continued production to focus on its development.

Aikido 合気道

Aikido was founded by Morihei Ueshiba (1883-1969), who was given the title of O-sensei (great teacher), which was a title of the founder of one of budo sports. As child was Ueshiba sickly and weak, and therefore he decided to train his body in the traditional martial arts such as judo, kendo (Japanese sword art), bojutsu (training with Lance), etc. The tough and purposeful training made him strong and physically fit. In his eagerness to reach the perfection began he to go hiking on the traditional way of the entire Japan, apart from one to the other and tested his skills against the famous champion. If any master was him superior he asked to get the stay as a student of his. When he taught himself everything that there was to learn in a place he pulled on. His technique honed and a day was counted he as one of the nation's leading in the traditional martial arts. Above all was he in 20 years ' time a pupil to Sokaku Takeda, who was of Samurai family and taught in jujutsu style Daito-Ryu Aikijujutsu. Ueshiba received coach license in Dai-to-ryu, and it is this martial art that had major influences in modern Aikido. In addition to training in different materiel arts, was Ueshiba greatly influenced by philosophical and religious of an abbot, Onisaburo Deguchi, who was the leader of a Japanese Shinto sect Omoto-kyo that was aimed against passivism and who wanted to build up a new society where Ueshiba during a number of years participated.

Ueshiba took part as a soldier 1902-1903 in Russia-Japanese war and in Macuriet in 1905. Through his martial arts training was he appointed to instructor in army of fight man by man. Ueshiba trained in military schools, among other things military police in budo. These experiences and influences from the religious sect Omoto-ryu brought about a change in Ueshiba view of budo sport. In connection with the second World War (1939-1945) in which Japan participated, so moved Ueshiba from Tokyo to the small village of Iwama where he completed his creation of aikido in its own new dojo (training hall). He introduced the new name Aikido for their martial arts style and straightforward techniques so that became a style without competition and where we make use of own force, not by blocking, but by controlled steer away the attacks.

His son Kisshomaru Ueshiba had after the war started on the dojo in Tokyo as Morihei Ueshiba earlier pushed and a organization named Aikikai as systematizes a grading system and marketed Aikido international. After Morihei Ueshiba died in 1969, so did his student Morihiro Saito (1928-2002) who was Ueshiba oldest pupil and Assistant to take over the Dojo in Iwama (see Figure 4.3).

Saito chose to preserve Ueshiba Aikido just so that he himself had to learn it, the style which today is known as Takemusu Aikido. Today, there are several styles of Aikido which formed by former students of Morihei Ueshiba as e.g. Ki-Aikido from Koichi Tohei or Hokuo Aikikai from Shoji Nisho.

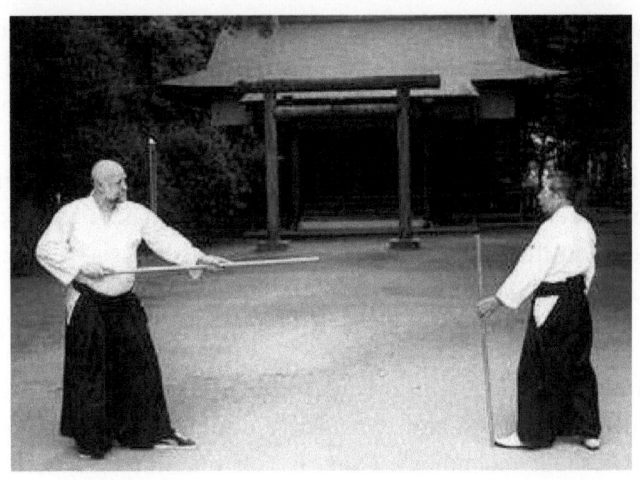

Fig. 4.3 Sensei Morihiro Saito 8 Dan, Ulf Evenås in Iwama dojo.
Photographer: Jöran Fagerlund

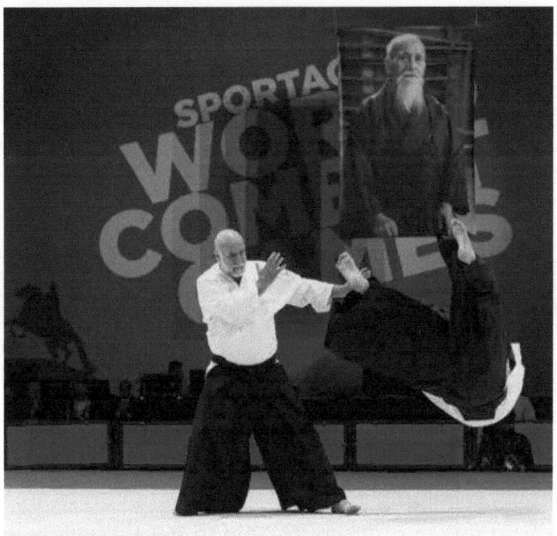

Fig. 4.4 Ulf Evenås 7 Dan, display World combat games 2013.
Photographer: Viktor Kazarin

I have been practicing Aikido in Göteborg Aikido club (dojo) which started in 1969 and still after 43 years, a booming business. The Club is run by Shihan Ulf Evenås 7 Dan who for many years took part in training for Saito in Iwama and during many seminars that Saito conducted in Europe. After Saito's death in 2002, so was named Ulf to leader of Takemusu Aikido in Europe. Ulf Evenås is very internationally hired for training camps in countries as Russia, Lithuania, Denmark, Germany, Australia and others and participated with display in "World Combat Games" held in St Petersburg 2013 (see Figure 4.4.)

Aikido training contains no element of competition, but because technicians carried out two and two, where one act attacking (Uke) and the other carries out technology (Nage). You practice each technique with both left and right arm, and then change the role of Uke and Nage. In more advanced stages are trained techniques where several Uke attacks with more dynamism and Nage must master to control off each attack.

Then many techniques in Aikido is derived from sword technology, so include your workout also training in sword techniques (Buki-Wasa) where a wooden sword (bokken) were used and different catas are carried out. Also training with a wooden stick (Jo) that was used by some martial arts schools in Japan are included as training. Sword technics is included for that give sense of distance and movement patterns to help get an understanding of, and facilitates regular Aikido training.

In Aikido, there is a rating system with different levels of ability named 6 kyu... 1 kyu and 1 Dan ... 8 Dan. As a beginner you start with grading to 6 kyu meaning to a number of static techniques (go tai), which starts by the attacker have a steady hold of for example the arm. During the later degrees coached technology in motion (the tai) where technology is started just before the attack is completed and in the higher degrees are trained to lead the attack on (ryu tai) in order to be able to get the attack under control. The thoughts is learning how a solid foundation that enables the representatives also works when you are under pressure and in the end leads to you the entire time can perform new techniques that suits the situation, in an endless flow.

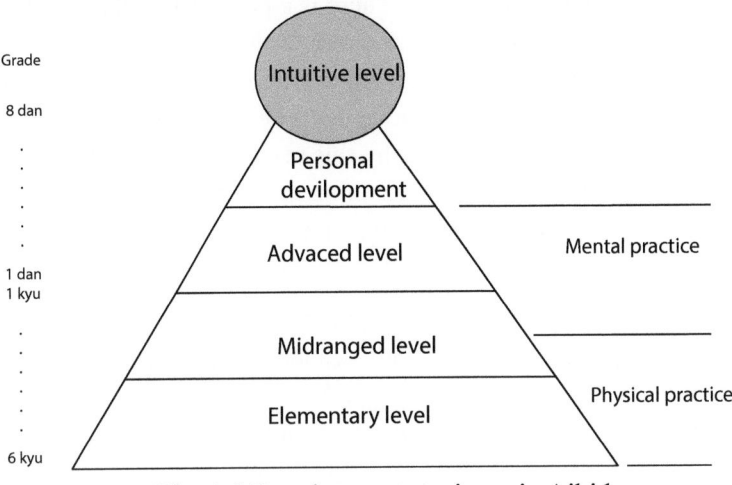

Fig. 4.5 Development staricase in Aikido.

Aikido and other martial arts have both a physical and a mental aspect of performance of techniques. In figure 4.5 shows a schematic picture how it develops in the different levels of knowledge and intuition, which correspond to levels in the rating system. In the elementary level are included to teach itself how the various technologies carried out physical, followed by the performance of the techniques in a reflective manner. In the higher levels do you train up the intuition so that intuitive implements appropriate technology against several attackers in an uninterrupted flow.

Through the systematic Aikido training so built a library up in the part of the brain that control fine motor skills in the body (cerebellum). This body consciousness that is available immediately, without mental conscious thoughts, gives that in a pressing situation in which one becomes infected not be paralyzed but instinctively steering away from the attack. You can see the Aikido training in light of Zen-do that to train up his instinctive and intuitive feeling so that the mind does not slow down the possible reaction in the prone position. The training means in addition to the physical activity while that to build up an internal sense of body consciousness as the Japanese call Ki. There is a point below the navel as the Japanese called " seika no itten" (the only point) that you can say is the body's Center of gravity where it says that Ki power emanates from. In Aikido practice it all the time to all movements because is in this point and to maneuver so that own power is led by this center. Some Aikido styles like for example Ki-Aikido has special training in order to build up a strong Ki power. At regular Aikido training you feel that this power be trained up and to move itself around its center even in mundane tasks.

In Aikido training includes also to practice breathing techniques, where in and exhaling synchronized with rendered techniques. Both weapons training and technique training use KIAI whereby a powerful sound screamed while making a technique is performed. The sound was used both to influence the attacker psychologically and to give more power to the executed technology. Aikido training also means that body consciousness immediately determines the possible attacker's intentions and in the best case, a planned attack averted in the early stages.

It is a number of scientific studies of how aikido training affects the practitioner, on the one hand, with measurable improvements in factors such as reaction time from external stimuli and both methods for to take advantage of the philosophical "non-violent" method for example management.

In the study "Six months aikido training shortens reaction time" of researchers Baris Sentuna, G Babayigit Irez, etc. (see ref. 4.1) has a number of aikido practitioners tested with respect to reaction times on external stimuli. The study's purpose is described: "a short reaction time is essential for aikido training. The intention of the study was to see what effect aikido training has on reaction times in a simple external stimuli or in a choice situation of a beginners and experienced practitioners. The study included 64 aikido practitioners aged 18-24 years with both men and women's. In preparation included, among other things the participants abstained from alcohol, smoking and coffee for at least 24 hours before the test was conducted. Participants training were exclusively aikido and no other sports.

Participants in the first group (34 people) were selected from a recently launched group of beginners in aikido. The other group (28 persons) had been practicing aikido between 6 months to 2 years before the test was performed. Tre different test connections with various aids were made for the dominant arm and the non-dominant arm. The first test was carried out by the person would push down a button with the index finger as soon as a lamp was lit and the reaction time was measured up. Test two was made in similar way but with a beep instead. Test 3 marked the choice between two stimuli before the press was made. Results of the study showed that aikido training improved both the reaction time of visual and audio stimuli and even decision-making time in choice situations was positively affected by regular aikido training.

As mentioned in the beginning of the chapter, so believe many that body consciousness is the body's sixth sense of perception. In many texts from the former champion in budo sport as described how after many years of training in a budo has built up a sensitivity in the body-consciousness that gives an intuitive perception of "danger" independent of conscious-ness and thus , an immediate reaction control away and prevent any attack. To exemplify how body consciousness seems like a sixth sense, so is budo sport of Ninjutsu that example, then one of the graduation to 5 Dan (Good) degree in this martial arts test of body consciousness.

Ninjutsu

Budo ninjutsu has become known pretty late in the 1970s in Europe on the basis of that in Japan has long been kept secret and only a small circuit ninjas have had access to the teaching of initiated masters. In Swe-den ninjutsu was introduced by Bo Munthe who comes into contact with Dr. Masaaki Hatsumi who is the 34 e grand master of the style Togakure Ryu, who is the last champion in a tradition since 800 years back in time. Hatsumi has inherited ancient ninjutsu-documents from his teacher, there different methods and abilities been preserved from the 800 year old tra-ditional teaching. In the book "Ninjutsu history and tradition" writes Hat-sumi: "Ninjutsu was developed as a counterculture against to the ruling

Samurai class and for the sake is the history hidden behind centuries of mystery, secrets and deliberate confusion".

You can compare the ninjas function in Japan with the secret organizations as the CIA in the United States and the KGB in the Russia in today's Western European societies. Ninja was hired for that infiltrate enemy camps and identify weaknesses in the opponent's defense. In both cases, the aim is to be the opponent shall be completely unaware of spy operations and take advantage of technologies to keep the operations.

Hatsumi describes ninjas role thus: "because of ninjas primary role as advisers, scouts and consultant to the days fighting foresees, got knowledge about espionage, psychological estimates and occult "sixth sense" forces prevail in front of fighting techniques for the battlefield. Despite to the historical Ninja was known as accomplished and merciless fighter was the nature of their work is usually such that if they must engage in combat for self-protection, it meant that their mission was automatically reduced in efficiency depending on that they had been discovered. Because this reason was ninjas arms usually regarded as backup measures in case of failure and not as the primary means of efficiency that previously were the case with Samurai ".

In ninjas education trained abilities in eighteen different areas, on the other hand, normal workouts in Taijutsu (punch, kick, grips , etc.) and different weapon techniques (sword, spear, missile , etc.) and part of the techniques in that able to infiltrate the enemies, masking, stealth and climbing techniques, explosives and blinding technics. As described earlier in this chapter to Zen-do is the mental attitude in budo, so write Hatsumi in his book: "Throw about to get to know effects and the influence of the body's many supply system can Ninpo eleven develop a working knowledge of his own forces for control of health and fitness in their body. The head is only one part of the body, and we must learn to overcome the tendency to distinguish between the brain and the body's other organ access. The body knows how it should be if we allow it to do so, and it does not need to be controlled with thought to react properly in a threatening situation. Ninpo eleven is working to eliminate the unnecessary process to first think through a response before action ". Because Ninja where out in the immediate vicinity or among the enemy, so trained Ninja to behave in such a way as to blend in with the surroundings and intuitive feel of any threat. In the higher degrees than ninjutsu trained body consciousness to intuitive feel of potential threats and for graduation from 4 Dan (Yodan) to 5 Dan (Godan) carried out an item that is called sakki (murder aura) or the test of truth.

The test is carried out by the aspirant sitting relaxed in the seiza position on the floor with closed eyes and a appointed sensei with higher Dan grade (e.g. Hatsumi) stand behind with raised swords (bamboo host) and suddenly makes a lunge toward the aspirants head. If the aspirant is aware of the attack and rolls away to the side without to be hit, is the test approved and 5 Dan level obtained. If the sword hit the head (very painful) is the test fail and further training must to for to be able to grade to 5th Dan. You call the test "murder aura" because we believe that if the battle meets someone who intends to kill someone, sends that person an energy called murder aura and that of a trained person can be understood of body consciousness. Those who have undergone the test mentions that in order to succeed one has to empty his mind from thoughts and be in a Zen state in which the mind is completely still. If you have reached the right state of mind, you instinctively an impulse to avoid the sword set in the right moment.

Israeli Doron Novon was the first non-Japan who trained ninjutsu for sensei Hatsumi under 6 years (1968-1974). Doron Novon started a dojo in ninjutsu budo after returning to Israel in 1974. Doron was the first Westerner who passed the sakki test in 1983 and obtained graduation 5 Dan (Godan).

Body consciousness as the sixth sense is also treated by the Morihei Ueshiba in the book: "The art of peace" (Ref. 4.3), Ueshiba had experience of Russia-Japanese war (1902-1903) and during a tough trip to Mongolia where he followed an abbot, Onisaburo Deguchi, who was the leader of the Japanese Shinto sect Omoto-kyo would proselytize for the sect and establish itself there. The trip ended in a total failure after that the group survived flood, hailstorms, poisoned food, near starvation, pirate's attacks and bombardment of Chinese army. The Group was sentenced to execution, but was saved in last moment of Japanese diplomacy. Ueshiba changed by these head-to-head mortal combat with murder pirates. In the book describes Ueshiba body consciousness saved him in vulnerable situations: "When we were in Tungliao were we duped into in a valley and were shot at by rifle bullets. Miraculously, I could feel the bullet paths, by rays of light indicated its courses and I could avoid the bombardment. Insight to be feel of an attack is it that previous budo masters mentions as being able to anticipate the event. If a person's mind is still and clean you can instinctively sense an attack and avoid it. I realized that this is the purpose of AIKI (the art of harmonization) ".

From the perspective of "The Unconscious Zone" have we in this chapter found that body consciousness is a source of fundamental power in the brains unconscious perception. Active training of budo or other sports affects reaction time for responses to external stimuli in a positive way. Some of these effects depends on that one through your workout more intuitive can take relevant decisions without the slower consciousness. In addition, after many years of training you intuitively perceive signs of "danger" and take appropriate action faster. As we will to see in the next chapter you can also in the "gut feeling" (body-mind) get intuitive indications that can save people from imposed dangers for example in the world of work.

Chapter 5 Intuition

The unconscious intelligence

Anyone who has ever engaged in creative activities such as graphic design, watercolor painting, research or design of electronics end up in thought patterns where you have hard to see the entire solution on the problem you have brought on themselves to solve. Despite that you set up in the heart of all parts and practically around with different hypotheses have been deadlocked in which ideas to solution has run out. It is often when you total trailer per at the solution and for example take a walk, meditate or take a vacation day that you suddenly see the solution in a night dream, or when you get a sudden inspiration when you were doing something else.

Many famous scientists have told us that when he reached for example new beyond the laws of physics, refers to his intuition where he suddenly see the whole solution on the problem as he explored unsuccessfully for a long time with his rational thinking.

Many quotes have been attributed to Albert Einstein, relativity author, which pronounced itself in many different topics in addition to science. When it comes to intuition, there is the following quote by Einstein: "The intuitive mind is a sacred gift and the rational mind is a faithful servant. We have created a society that celebrates the servant and lost away the gift".

Another physicist that formulated electromagnetics famous Maxwell's equations (1865), was James Clerk Maxwell who on his death bed on intuition spoke: "That is made of it which is called I, is probably made of something in me that is greater than I".

If you turn up the word intuition in encyclopedia (NE) says that:"Intuition, the ability to immediately perceive something, in which case all elements perceived direct, without support of the experience or intellectual analysis. The majority of analytical philosophers reject the idea of such a irrational way of knowledge".

Psychotherapist Carl G Jung writes in his book man and his symbols: "sensations are talking about for us that something can be found, the thinking informs us about what it is, the feeling will determine if it pleases us or not, the intuition is talking about the forms of the will and where it leads".

What is meant with the word intuition is not clearly defined between different researchers, philosophers, or in the "new age". In the continued description, a number of different approaches and models subjected to screening for brain's handling of unconscious processes that are included in "The Unconscious Zone". In psychology, it has been in recent decades made great progress in research into how our minds dealing with incoming perception from our five senses. Among other things, with the help of modern magnetic resonance equipment (fMRI) carefully has been able to map different areas in the brain, where specific interaction occurs at different types of experiment studies of the brain. Through controlled experiments, one can identify the different processes that characterize the intuitive (unconscious) thinking.

System1 respective system 2

The two psychologists Keith Stanovich and Richard West are some of the pioneers of Psychology who conducted research on the processes involved in our thinking launched in a report (year 2000) the designations system1 and system 2 for it automatically unconscious thinking and the conscious respective the rational intellectual tasks. Just intuition is associated with system1, there the brain immediately in real time unconsciously automatically processes incoming sensory input. Where it either directly controls on for example routine driving or when you instinctively pulls away your hand about to burn itself. While it alarm system 2 when you need to process incoming stimuli with logical considerations and decisions. Stanovich and West define how the brain works in a "Dual process" according to:

• System 1: Is an unconscious processing (process type 1) that works automatically and quickly via parallel processing of senses with large capacity and where normal consciousness do not experience any conscious control.

• System 2: Is the processing (process type 2) which we are normally aware of and where you think they have control by concentration and can make conscious choices. Typically experience a particular effort in connection with the intellectual activities such as more complex mathematical calculations, where between results maintained in working memory.

The theories about the thought processes that affect system 1 or system 2 have become widely accepted in the psychological research. Keith Stanovich and Jonathan Evans are debating an article ("Dual-process theories of higher cognition; Advancing the debate ", 2013, ref. 5.1) objections from other researchers against the theory of "dual-processes" and considers that recent research supports this theory of two processer. In the item's summary notes Stanovich and Evans to system 2 supports hypothetical thinking and put stress on working memory hard. While system 1 which is a fast automatic process adopted and could leave faulty interpretation of sensory input if it does not become controlled by system 2.

In table 5.1 shows an overview of the typical features of the system 1 respective system 2:

Type 1 process	Type 2 process
Intuitive	Reflective
Need not working memory	Using working memory
Automatic	Mental stimulation
Fast	Slow
High capacity	low capacity
Unconscious	Conscious
Parallel	Serial
Distorted	Normative
Contextual	Abstract
Automatic	Controlled
Associative	Rule based
Experiment based decision	Consequence based decision
Regardless of the possible perception	Correlated perception

System 1 (older brain function)	System 2 (newer brain function)
Earlier development	Evolution
Similar to animal processing	Unique human processing
Implicit knowledge	Explicit Knowledge
Basic emotion	Complex emotion

Table 5.1

Professor emeritus at Princeton University's Daniel Kahneman received the Economics Prize to Alfred Nobel's memory in 2002, has in a book "think fast and slow", 2013 (ref. 5.2), development theories regarding system 1 and system 2. Kahneman who worked on psychological intuition at Hebrew University in Jerusalem collaborated with Amos Tversky (from 1969) who worked with decision research. Cooperation during a 15 -year period resulted in a number of high-profile articles on intuitive judgments and decision making under risk.

A way for the reader to experience how the two systems are working , will be shown with two simple experiments.

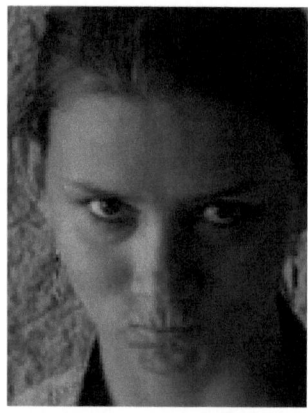

Look at the first picture 5.1 for a short while.

Already after a short glance starts your intuitive thinking and you have lightning quick reading of the image and can probably explain a number of intuitive impressions. The person sees angry out and will for sure to attack someone verbally. This is an example of system 1 way to subconsciously scan the surrounding area and notify the system 2 an intuitive perception.

To activate the system 2 required more complex considerations, for example a mathematical problem. If we are asked what is 2 + 2 =? We have certainly a quick intuitive answer, but if you give a more complicated calculation task needs to engage the system 2 and thereby enable working memory. A calculation of the expression 25x18 =? Calls for normal to you make a multiplication shelf which contains intermediate result before the total calculation is ready. You can probably quickly give a range within which the result is located (for example, 25x20 = 500; 25x10 = 250) but the end result 450 requires probably paper and pen.

Kahneman and Tversky research came to focus on the study of how distortions (Bias) occurs and affects the intuitive thinking of system 1. Through a series of psychological experiments identified a twenty speech mechanisms that provide distortion (systematic error) in intuitive judgement. The results were presented in an article in the journal Science titled "Judgment under uncertainty: Heuristics and biases" see ref. 5.3. The article was noticed much in the scientific community and has influenced many areas as medical diagnose, legal judgement, IQ test, philosophy, etc. This to point on mechanisms witch can unconsciously influence the result in research or decision making.

Kahneman and Tversky comes through experiments up to three different typesofheuristics(rulesofthumb)whounwittinglymightreducecomplexrelationshipsofprobabilityandpredictionstomorestraightforwarddecision-making criteria which can distort the results of assessments made by system 1.

• Representativeness

• Accessibility

• Anchoring, alignment

From the represent point of view, identified a number of parameters that you unconsciously can be overlooked from for example previous probability calculations, the size of the sample, the measurement's validity, according probability, and misunderstanding of randomness.

Distortions on the basis of availability are affected by e.g. how frequently there have been easy-to-access data, imagination and illusory correlation.

Anchoring effect: give a specific value to an unknown quantity before estimated and adjustment is affected by whether it is initially located far from the expected value.

As an example of how a process is created for anchorage describes an experiment Kahneman which Realtors would value a House that was already laid out for sale. They visited the House and got read a rich booklet about the House, which also contained information about the asking price. Half of the agents got to see a requested price that was much higher than that requested, while half see a requested price that was much lower. Every broker had set a reasonable price for the House and a minimum price that could be accepted. Agents had to give an account of the factors which influenced the assessment. Curiously, heard the asking price are not the factors, without brokers made a point that they did not take account of it. They were convinced on to the requested price not influenced their answer, but they were wrong in this point. Anchoring effect of brokers was 41 % while a respective group of students ended up at 48 percent.

A consequence of anchors effect is that in a negotiation about the price of dealing, so is it the who first put an anchor value that controls the final valid price.

At summery can Kahneman/Tversky research on system 1 (Intuitive impression) and system 2 (logical considerations) in some general descriptions.

System 1 (Intuitive impression) is an early developed systems to continuously receive and analyze the impression that affects an individual's survival. Questions could be as how it looks out into the surrounding area right now, are it something worrying threat or opportunity that cannot be missed, feels any of-receding scent, hear any unusual noises or is everything normal. Continuous reports of threat scenarios are given to system 2. Signals are given to move closer or pulling itself away, rate the impression that good or bad and trigger decision to flee or stay. System 1 response is controlled by previous experiences where more recent events and context weighs most heavily, and thereafter older memories have importance. In this context plays associative memory a large role, which often several different impressions can be activated coherent, where for example fragrance, audio and visual together provides an associative memory. Associative memories triggered by e.g. a certain smell that directly via the limbic system triggers a complex image that is associated with this particular event. The advantage with system 1 quick conclusions is to relieve system 2 with routine decision where it is controlled by "spinal cord feeling". While the neck part is that it may make irrevocable choices, without knowledge to be aware of that. These decisions can be inaccurate or poorly informed. Phobias of various kinds, for example snake horror is often associated with flashbacks where an accident or dangerous situation stored in the associative memory. This can induce unwarranted fear just by seeing a stick lying on the forest path.

Another unconscious influence of system 1 is prajming (subliminal influence), which is an effect which unconsciously influenced in their decisions, for example words, pictures or advertisements that you observed without being aware of them. Prajming turn off the associated ideas network and brings the Association courts in accordance with the prajming content. System 1 draw quick conclusions and is more uncritical to distortions and biases than the system 2 and more susceptible to mood swings that make the person less vigilant and prone to commit logical mistakes.

System 2 (logical considerations) generally have a lower capacity than calculation system 1, but possesses the ability to strenuous intellectual activities that require attention. If system 1 does not have a quick answer to a question is activated system 2 which focuses attention and looking for in memory after answer. System 2 uses working memory for intermediate results and makes complex calculations, compare, plan and select out logical solutions or decisions. System 2 also have a supervisory function over results from system 1, system 2 approves the proposal, giving the impression, intentions to beliefs and convey impulses to act, which also take account of self-control. System 2 also works after through-pass tasks with minimal effort. Generally impair a fast-paced and stress thoughts ability in system 2. When system 2 works consumed much glucose in the brain, which is why we at intellectual work can feel tired and have to add sugar.

Intuitive decisions

Gary Klein is in the United States active psychology researchers that interest for the experts make intuitive decisions in environments where quick decisions have to be taken in occupations as fire officers, emergency nurses or helicopter pilots and where decisions often comes to life or death. Klein argues that research in these areas must be made directly in the environment in which decisions are taken and cannot replace by experiments in a laboratory environment where the pressure of time and results do not have the same essential.

Klein started 1978 its own company Klein Associates Ltd. which was in directed towards research in how decisions are made out of real often time-pressed environment. The company received a contract from the U. S. Army Research institute in 1984 with the mission to examine how decisions are made by experts in extremely time critical circumstances and where decisions affect liv, death and damage of buildings. The work resulted in a technical report (Technical Report 796, 1988, Rapid Decision Making on the fire ground, ref. 5.4) directed to the originator U. S. Army Research institute as outgoing from the report implemented the proposed model (RPD) in Arm instructions for policy management in command/control centers.

Klein decided that an appropriate group of experts to study was fire officers who are responsible for that lead staff and manage resources at fire-places and other accidents where the Fire Department is alarmed. The study interviewed 26 fire officers with long experience of fire-fighting (in average years of experience in the profession 23.2). In-depth interviews were made on 32 critical accidents of varying process and focused questions on how fire officers took their decision at the arrival to the scene of the accident. The researchers identified 156 decision-making occasions of which 132 in one minute time frame.

When the study began, the researchers assumed that fire commanders took the decision according to the standard deductive logical process in which a number of options was through before a decision on how the fire would be addressed. When Klein asked a fire officer about the decision he had taken, he got a quizzical look and told "I have not taken any decision". Klein identified that fire officers not listed a number of options that would be reviewed, but made an overall assessment of how the entire fire situation looked like and immediately conjured up a recollection of the experience from the many hundred previous fires with similar appearance that he attended. The researchers called this a prototype and thus decided to fire command intuitively measures according to the usual methods applicable for this fire case. Off the 156 decision-making opportunities so touched 127 of the decisions dealing with such a prototype fire. This decision-making method means that no conscious examination is made; instead an immediate recognition of patterns (fire type) was made and fighting started then immediately according to the usual routines. Fire Officer asked the question "What happens" on arrival to the fire place and a number of impressions are analyzed in seconds about if there are open fire, smoke, intensity etc.

In the report describes Klein about a case where the fire command himself believed that he had taken the decision as the result of an ESP (extrasensory perception) experience, which Klein was able to analyze and explain as a consequence of the expert's experience.

The crew comes out to a fire at the back of a House. Fire command assesses that there is a fire in the kitchen and provide firefighters with water hose for extinguishing in the kitchen. Though pouring with water is not the fire subsides in the normal way and fire officer standing in the living room will be baffled by the fire increased intensity in spite of water diffusion. The firemen retreat for to regroup. Fire Officer got an unpleasant feeling that fire events were not normal and ordered fire-men to quickly pull themselves back. Within a minute, collapsed the floor in the House down in the basement and had brought with it danger for firefighters ' lives if they remained inside. Afterwards realized fire command to fire events did not happen according to his initial assessment of the fire. The fire turned out to be in the basement and thus affected the water diffusion not fire normally, the warmth of the living room was also elevated and normal sound from the fire was unusually low. It was this pattern that did not match that the fire officer experience with similar fires, bringing the intuitive decision on evacuation. Fire com-

mand believed that he had had an ESP experience who saved colleagues '
liv, while Klein identified that the underlying factors instead was that the
fire did not match past experience and thus evacuated the House quickly.

Klein's model of explanation of how the fire officer intuitive decision builds up involves a long period of time in which the experience of previous fires that stored in memory and how to successfully
fought fires. This is an implicit learning and when you are faced with
a new fire so looking to intuitive after a match against former experienced fires. Senior fire officer has a whole set of past fire events stored
which will help to solve how the attack should be designed, while
a new firefighter will need the help of the rules to know what to do.

The method involves a singular activity where you do not compare different options without identifying a likely possible approaches
and evaluates the exportability of success and choose direct task if it is
thought to clear the task even if the method is not optimal. If your command does not quickly find a prototype case, so start a mental simulation
where he represents what consequences a supposed scenario would have.
If the result of simulating seems adequate are the activity implemented
otherwise rejected scenery and a new mental simulation is carried out.

In the report identified Klein a model for decision making that instead of to analyze a number of parallel alternatives which then is
compared to the choice of approach in figure 5.1, so managing fire officers an approach where a similar prototype fire and quickly found
with mental simulation of method is adequate. Otherwise, elected a new proto-typical cases until they feel themselves happy with
the likely outcome (see Figure 5.2), after which the fire is attacked

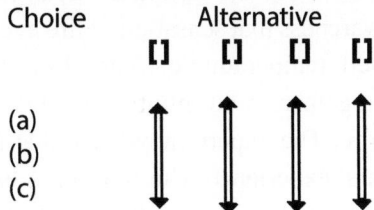

Figur 5.1 Alternative choice

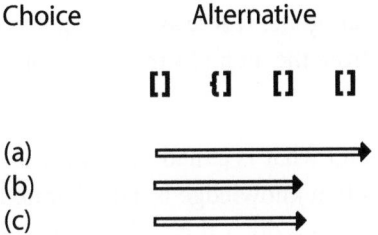

Figur 5.2 Sequence choice

In the report gives a decision model: Recognition-Primed Decision modell see fig. 5.3.

Fig. 5.3 Recognition-Primed Decision Modell (RPD)

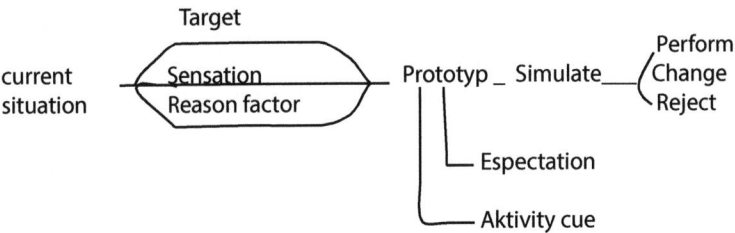

The most important decision point is to ask the question "What happens" and get an accurate situational awareness that sensation of fire events from all the senses (sight, hearing, smell, temperature etc.) and from any witness people on site by weighting together to an intuitive impression in order to choose the right porotype fire. The expert knowledge that fire officers use based on 10, 15 or 20 years' experience who built up a base of patterns (fire type) as a result of the quick decisions that need to be done can be done in an intuitive way. This intuitive decision taken partly unconsciously by system 1, but need to be monitored by system 2, so no obvious mistake committed. The other important factor is expectations on how made measures on the current fire has gone, where system 2 can verify that the selected prototype fire process from the mental simulation conform to current mode.

The intuition is about competence and what is called tacit knowledge, which is taught in implicit, whereas explicit knowledge is a deliberate factual knowledge. Silent knowledge is , among other things if our ability to take in all the sensations associated with a given event, the ability to pattern recognition, ability to see abnormalities in the typical pattern and that we have mental models of how things work.

The outcome in the described case with kitchen fire shows the fire officer first decision on prototype fire not correct, but when the results of the control are not followed the mental simulation, so was vacated the House, then fire command noted deviations from expected results.

Daniel Kahneman and Gary Klein have something different opinions regarding the intuitive decisions, among other things when Kahneman through a series of experiments shown on the risk of many types of distortions (Bias) from system 1 , which manages the intuitive message. An exchange of ideas between Kahneman and Klein regarding the perception of intuitive decisions during an 8 year period are published in a report, "Conditions for intuitive expertise: (a) failure to disagree" , see ref. 5.5. Kahneman argues that it must be a certain regularity in the environment to consider expert to be able to provide a safe estimate, but admits that in the fire officer cases so far as intuitive decision on basis of the extreme time pressure.

Quotes from Albert Einstein and James Clerk Maxwell in the chapter introduction matches the expert model with system 1 for intuitive and system 2 for rational judgement. When scientists make breakthrough in research to new physical lows, so is usually data collection over the decades and perhaps unsuccessful experiments behind a number of associative memories where you suddenly find intuitive pattern to the solution of the problems. Many times, a failed experiment are behind new discoveries that can be illustrated with the case where Ian Fleming found penicillin in an off-forgot sample in the lab, which led to the development of antibiotics for treatment of infection diseases.

Expert research

In this context, we mention the research subject expertise as the Swedish Professor in psychology at Florida State University Anders Ericsson has implemented. Ericsson studied how, among other things musician and chess-player was developed in their respective abilities to gaining expert knowledge. He wanted to find out if it is the common assumption about talent or innate predisposition that was the decisive property to achieve highly in their respective field of expertise.

Studies made at the Berlin Music Academy with an examination of the three groups violin pupils, where group one was composed of students who were considered to be soloists in world-class, group two of the students who were good and a third group which was thought to be a music teacher. Common was that everyone started playing violin in the 7 years of age, but in teens increasing the differences. At 20 year age group one had an accumulated over 10000 hours of exercise while group two practiced 8000 hours and group three 4000 hours. A corresponding amateur-musician is around 2000 hours of exercise in the same age. The study observed that some of the best pupils are trained from an early age 50-60 hours a week and that they exercised more alone (25 hours/week) than the ones that were considered a little less developed who trained individual 10 hours/week.

The researchers found that the main ingredient in the exercises was that the student had contact with a violin teacher of high class who always gave the student data as low on the level of what the student passed by (deliberate practice). Anders Ericsson noted that in order to reach the highest levels in music, so should we have trained at least 10000 hours and no students who have not exercised as much reached the top. It came up to be this type of exercise with a gradually increasing difficulty (deliberate practice) applied in other fields and even to an accumulated experience in 10000 hours required in order to get to a level of expertise in a business with fairly complex structure. To be effective training will be as practice related as possible.

Science journalist Malcolm Gladwell has in a book " the Outliners" studies factors behind that a person gets success and become high achievers. He notes that the social security account manager to context and environment is a key factor when a child grows up and, for example starts to play a musical instrument. If the student chooses something that arouses interest and environment is supportive and encouraging facilitated front steps, which are necessary to put down the 10000 hours it takes to be the soloist in the world. This is also a competent teacher who can provide progressively more difficult exercises to stimulate pupils learning.

Own experiences after 50 years of activity with design work and troubleshooting of complex computer-controlled real-time systems, among other things in flying radar stations for interceptor Viggen and the JAS project, pointing to that the intuitive systems1 plays a major role especially during problem solving. A development process starts with learning about what the design should cope with, which results in a requirement specification. Often during the progress of construction, you end up in situations where you do not know how the resulting problem must be solved , but after a time frustrated unsuccessful work with rational thinking, so POPs an intuitive spontaneous solution up to seemingly without intellectual effort. Especially for advanced troubleshooting of complex computer systems, get an experienced Troubleshooter Guide of the many previously resolved and corrected the errors in the various electronic systems that are stored in the associative memory.

In the majority of companies are people with silent knowledge that during decades implicitly built up a field of knowledge that often is invaluable in maintaining the company's survival, we call it often "to the knowledge sitting in the walls ". In the radio show "Car doctor" is the expert "Bosse car doctor" to answer listeners' questions about problems with their motors. Bosse which has 50 years of experience as a repairman asking questions about the possible sounds, fragrances or exhaust fumes for the encircling of error cause to solve the problem in similar way as fire officers earlier in the text, and can usually help listeners to grips with intuitive answers.

Intuition and body language

Another use of intuition is made of esterified artists who work as mentalist. They have shows where it reads the people from the audience and with help of his intuition "read people's thoughts" or affect the person to various unexpected behavior. One such artist is Fredrik Praesto operating in Sweden and who published a book on intuition (Intuition: a book on how you make use of your hidden resources 1997, Liber AB, ref. 5.6).

Praesto, originally trained as a construction engineer describes in the book how he through an intuitive sense survived a construction site accident and then went to a new work as illusionist and mentalist. In the book explain Presto initially for how he worked as a construction engineer in a construction bridge of Klarabers bridge in Stockholm. In Praesto job included, among other things to check the casting of the concrete portion on top of stamp towers that make up the bridge. After the concrete is pumped up in the wood form must to check that the bridge not falling unevenly during the drying process. Prestos job was to climb up in the towers and crawl into during the wooden molds with the setting concrete and read by a number of scales that would be reported to the Manager. At the first control was results approved. When he would make the next control felt he instinctively that he was not wanted there up, but the whole of his body from said "thou shalt not there up". He found in a number of other things that "must" be done first in order to pull out on time, but the time for that report to the Manager approached. He realized that it would not be well received if he spoke about his unpleasant feeling and ignore in that climb up. Just then heard a tremendous bang and wood form plummeted down as a House of cards and the concrete was crushed to the ground. An accident that cost millions but luckily no one was injured.

After an internal accident investigation it turned out that the carpenters who built the mold botched with number of nails that the drawings described. Praesto that appeared when the mold was built thinks he might unwittingly noticed that this two Carpenter's way to nail was different or he felt some vibrations in the stamp form which unconsciously influenced him. In analogy with the previously presented the case of the fire officer who evacuated the building before the floor collapsed, one can see the case of the cast stamp form. The intuitive unconscious factors that have seen are probably behind the decisions that saved lives in these two cases.

In his new role as a mentalist has Praesto honed his intuition to the feel of the body language from the people who he put up out of the audience at the scene shows. A number that often take place in the show is that five people are asked to draw their arbitrary figure on his sketchpad but that mentalist cannot see the figures. Then set the five paintings back and Praesto ask each person it is he who created the image and all must answer no. Praesto can then point out who made each figure with the help of the reactions that he picks up in body language. Another way to influence the subjects ' choices in a choice situation, is to display figures or numbers that volunteers subconsciously get through prajming, for selecting one of the mentalist predetermined value. The prajming figure can for example be in a number of images that are included in the show, but usually without mentioning it explicit. In the next chapter dealt with the topic how the unconscious body language affect us and can be used by mentalists and also by salesman in dealing situations.

In this chapter, a number of approaches and explanations are given on how intuition affects us in "The Unconscious Zone". It is a large unaware capacity in the brain that helps us to solve complex contexts and problems, which famous scientists often have declared that they use then discoveries were made. Experts in various fields have stored large amounts of previously problem solutions, which via intuition are quickly available for to solve current tasks or dissuade from previous failed performing.

It is important not to completely rely on intuition but system 2 should check the reasonableness of proposed measures when risk of various distortions in the system 1 can happen. In conjunction with intuition is talking to often on gut feeling that many believe is linked to the unconscious intuitive awareness of system 1. You talk about "butterflies in the stomach" when, for example faced with a task that you must keep a speech before a large audience. There is a strong connection between the stomach and the brain via the vagus nerve which connects a large number of internal organs with the brain. The enteric nervous system in the gut, known often as "the second brain", when it contains more than 100 million nerve cells that control the intestinal work and can signal to the brain about the status and possible stomach problems. In the crucial situations as to determine if new working place, new life partners and living environment, so think I it is necessary that your gut is not neglected, but that one is trying to understand the underlying causes of it. As the previous examples demonstrated, so can it in extreme cases safe the life. In the next chapter are the body language described as a source of perception, which often forms the basis of intuitive feelings and the influence of the decision.

Chapter 6 Body language

The unconscious communication

As people interact we every second with the surroundings and especially when we talk with other people in social context, as there are many unconscious signals in "The Unconscious Zone" as we catch up and that control our reactions on different ways. Already when we are small children so imitate we our parents and when they smile, so we automatically smile back.

Recent research by a group of Italian researchers under the direction of Giacomo Rizzolatti at the University of Parma, pointing out some neurons in the brain, called mirror neurons, which can be said to be behind the unique ability to human compassion (Article in Brain in 1996, ref. 6.1). The researchers studied monkeys (macaques) to measure how the brain controls the targeted movements, as to grab items, through to record signals from individual neurons in the motor part of the brain, when the monkey grabbed foods. At one of the experiments reached out to one of the researchers grabbed after a banana and at the same time reacted neurons in the monkey. The researchers were surprised by that the motor nerves that control muscles reacted on the monkey's sights. Further experiments showed that neurons gave similar signals when the monkey was performing a movement as if it was someone else makes a similar move. Even the sound when any other eats a peanut got the monkey's nerve cells to react as if he eats the peanut. Neurons in the monkey's brain simulated signals corresponding to the monkey himself performed the action.

The further research has shown that the human brain acts in a similar way, and it is larger areas with specialized mirror neuron in the human brain. The results indicate that, with the help of mirror neurons may put us in in other people's condition, which in the extension can mean that we can learn in advanced motor skills, by to consider other people. Attempts have been made with beginners in golf who had learning to golf, to see other players on computer screens playing golf and thus in the brain simulated the neural pathways involved in golf game.

In experiment have showed that mirror neuron can identify the intension with an act. Experiments with monkeys showed that there are different nerve cells that register a hand that moves an apple or a hand witch moves the apple towards the mouth of to eat. Researcher Christian Keyser's has identified that there are mirror neurons in the human brain that can reflect movements, intentions and pure emotions. He notes also that research has shown that the degree of empathy with a man may be linked to high activity in mirror neuron, which affects the degree of compassion of an individual. Mirror neurons have been to major research field, which proved that Brocas area of the brain, which control motor speech, contains many mirror neurons and is central to language learning in children. This may be an explanation for the child's language development when they first learn to speak by mimicking the movements of the face and mouth.

When it comes to body language is the most likely explanation for us in various situations mimics people we consider, for example yawn, laughing or reflecting body positioner, in activity in our own mirror neuron, that reflects the person's movements and feelings.

Facial expressions

Professor emeritus of psychology, Paul Ekman is one of the pioneers when it comes to understanding of body language in which he especially focused on facial expressions and gesture. Earlier considered the research that for example expressions of joy and sorrow was culturally conditioned and learned. Ekman decided to explore how indigenous peoples who have not had contact with Western culture expressed their feelings in corresponding situations and decided to go to Papua New Guinea 1967 and visit the Fore people who lived in the stone age level to study their non-verbal behavior. His theory was that as Darwin predicted, facial expressions are universal and partly congenital. Ekman filmed and recorded on tape how residents reacted in different manifestations of joy, fear and sorrow in situations that he staged. He had also a Gallery with pictures with portrait

151

of happy and sad Americans, where the inhabitants through the interpreter would explain their interpretation of emotions. Ekman's evaluation of the collected material showed that before people's faces in various situations correspond exactly with our own faces in the Western world. This gives that because the basic emotions like joy, sorrow, fear and anger is expressed as ubiquitous, they are innate.

Ekman's continued research focused on identifying all the possible facial expressions that can be developed by various muscles in the face and create a library for recognition of these facial expressions. Together with the researcher W Friesen created Ekman 1978 the first comprehensive tool to objectively measure facial movement which was given the name Facial Action Coding System (FACS). The system assigns each facial movement a number where for example. "9" means wrinkle your nose and "15" means squeezing the lips. A feeling can be expressed through to several facial movements are combined such as sorrow the expression 1 + 4 + 15, where "1" means inner eyebrow movement and "4" eyebrow reduction. The degree of expression is specified with a letter of A ... E where E is the maximum expression. Total is 46 different facial movements possible to enter and in addition, there are more number of head movements and position of the head. Out of body language point of view, these expressions are not normally under conscious control, but reflect the person's emotional state. The big emotions such as sorrow, joy and anger is expressed normally for longer periods of time from seconds to minutes and is called Macro expression.

Research in this area has focused on something that is called Micro expression. It has made recordings of faces during experiments in which the person knowingly to lie about certain things such as to have taken money from an envelope. The researchers were able in "slow motion" note that the subjects in connection with to the lied has transient expression in the face during parts of a second, typically 1/5 seconds, where we subconsciously shows what they really think of the question they lied about , for example disgust. Paul Ekman has systematized this research to training packages where border policemen and interrogators are trained to be able to recognize when suspects are lying by identifying Micro expressions in their faces. Trained interrogators reviewing video footage of the interview to identify Micro expressions by in "slow motion" during playback evaluate the suspect person. Evaluation of a 10-minute recording requires about three hours for an experienced interrogators.

An interesting development of the recognition of facial expressions made by Marian Stewart Bartlett who is professor at the University of California, San Diego and is a researcher at Institut for Neural Computer (UCDC). The research involves algorithms to recognize facial expressions according to Paul Ekman's mapping FACS. The Institute's research is focused on that in real time to evaluate natural communication such as visual, auditory, and tactile communication.

A number of projects are underway to realize computer algorithms in the following areas:

• Automatic interpretation of facial expressions in Facial Action Coding Systems (FACS).

• Automatic analysis and classification of liar according to FACS.

• Recognition and tracking of faces in real time.

• Recognition and tracking of certain diseases (e.g., autism).

• Automatic speech recognition.

• Social robots for classroom learning.

Research on the automatic registration of facial expressions is funded by the defense originations "Homeland Security" in the United States and the results are expected to be used by interrogators and guards at airports in the United States. Already, there are computer programs with similar evaluation results of liars who experienced interrogators have. Further research is going on there, by means of an infrared camera can identify hot spots in the face during interrogation and see changes among other things around the eyes when the person lies. Research where you combine a regular camera with an IR camera to further enhance the security of to assess if someone is lying is done via computer fusion where they both bulletins are correlated.

The research has resulted in that it identified seven basic emotions: sorrow, joy, fear, anger, disgust, surprise and contempt which one can express in different degree by, among other things speaking, facial expressions, Micro expressions, gesture, looking, posture and tone of voice. The library over possible facial expression contains about 10000 different combinations of which about 3000 are included in natural behavior and about 100 are used in a normal conversation. Out of body language's point of view is the interpretation of facial expressions a source to read of what a person really thinks and very useful for e.g. mentalist when in the shows read of the Micro expressions contributors to "read their thoughts".

Body language is also a cultural dimension which it e.g. can interpret gestures differently in different countries. Also the close comfort zone can vary greatly, as in India, where it is much closer to the people you talk with than in for example the Nordic countries. Researcher Edward Hall introduced in 1966, the term "proxemics" for the study of the natural distance between the people who interact with each other. He identified four different distances as in the West, reveals the relationship between the people involved in the talks.

• An intimate distance of approx. 50 cm is reserved for lovers, child or close family members and friends.

• Personal distance is between 50 cm and 1.2 m and is turned in talking to friends, colleagues or group discussion.

• Social distance varies from about 1.2 m to 2.4 m and reserved for strangers, newly formed groups and new friends.

• Public distance varies from about 2.4 m to 8 m and is used in speeches, lectures and theater.

If you come for near the intimate distance at meeting with a stranger, it can be perceived as aggressive behavior and results often in discomfort in the face of the situation. One other aspect that affects body language can be conditioned by the conventions of a specific country, where people such as in Italy is used to express himself sweeping in discussions, while in Japan are ideal to mask their feelings public by politely smile and bow in many situations.

Body language significance

In newspapers and articles regarding body language indicates it is often that the relationship between how we communicate with each other is 55 % with the body, 38% with the voice and just 7 % of the words. Researcher Albert Merahbian (professor emeritus in psychology) who in a report 1967 entered these numbers has strongly denied that this would apply generally for body language. The current report concerned the experiment where he knowingly made assertions where body language and/or tone of voice did not match the spoken words. Albert Merahbian found that the verbal component of regular communication was about 35% and non-verbal about 65 % of communication. A note can be it must vary big time for example a clown or mime artist using near 100% body language, while a complex lecture in mathematics or physics emphasizes the concepts of verbal communication.

A popularization of body language during the 1970s was initiated by the author Julius Fast through the publication of the book "body language", 1970, see ref. 6. 2. One of the notable findings was how John Kennedy defeated Richard Nixon in the presidential campaign in the United States in 1960. A new component in the election campaign was to debates in television between the candidates came to play a crucial role in John Kennedy's favor. It turned out that those who followed the debate via radio had Nixon as won the debate, while those who watched the debate on television had

Kennedy as the winner. Kennedy had a better body language while Nixon was sweating profusely and looking unkempt out with dithering look, saw Kennedy cool, elegant and secure out with a fixed gaze. Clear had body language a crucial importance in TV media. A similar process took place during the presidential campaign between Jimmy Carter and Gerald Ford in 1976. In the first debate won the Gerald Ford while Carter won the second debate by media advisers who trained in fixed gaze, more open posture, more certain gestures and better voice control. During the elections in 1976 in Sweden there was a similar effect where a major election debate in the Scandinavium in Göteborg between Olof Palme and Thorbjörn Fälldin came to affect the outcome of the elections. Present at the debate in the Scandinavium arena felt that Palme had won the debate, while the large viewers as seen on TV debate felt that Palme had a body language that was arrogant and nasty while Fälldin which was noticeably nervous and sweated got viewers ' sympathies. For today's politicians included media training including body language and PR agencies to provide maximum impact of special TV audience in debater.

Conscious influence of body language

An interesting aspect about the body language has been identified by the researcher Amy Cuddy worked as Associate Professor at the Harvard Business School and who has a doctorate in social psychology from Princeton University. Cuddy is known for his research on discrimination, stereotype, emotion and power at non-verbal behavior (body language) and its impact on the body's hormone levels, such as testosterone and cortisol. In a report in the journal Psychological Science 21, 2010 sets out for experiments with person who tested for risky behavior and may be subject to a staged interview. The experiments were conducted under two different conditions in which the subjects in one case under 2 minutes before the attempt would adopt postures that involve power with a straight back and dominant posture. In other case would the subject take a subordinate position for 2 minutes before the experiment with Crouching posture with crossed arms (see Figure 6.1, 6.2).

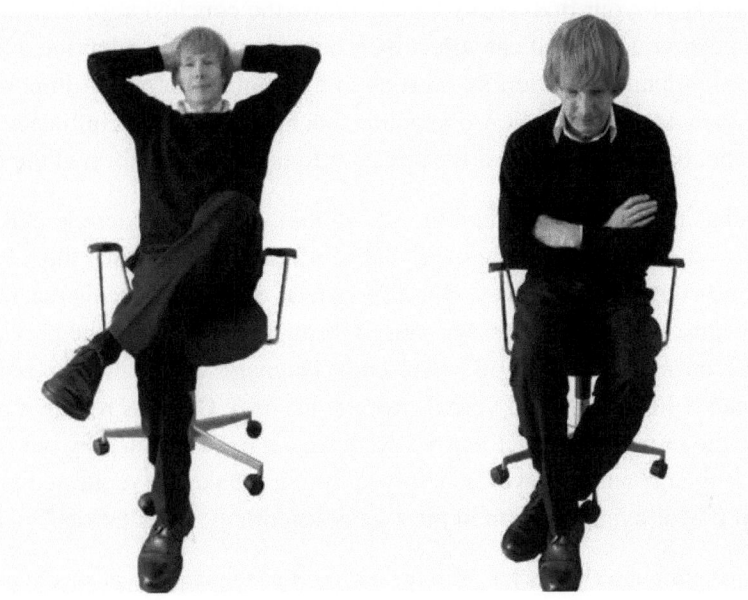

Fig 6.1 Dominant body language. Fig. 6.2 Subordinate body language

The subjects made first a test where we judged how risky they were. Of the persons who before the test had found themselves in the power of dominant condition proved to be 86% take risk, while those who took an under-arranged role before the test so was 60 % take risk. The subjects were also subject to a staged interview during the 5 minutes. The interviewer would not provide any feedback to the subject during the interview and the test was carried out under stress. Consistently held respondents to the subjects who had taken a dominant state prior to the interview were those who would have received job offers. When they measured hormone levels for the two categories of subjects so testosterone increased by 20% for the dominant and the decreased by 25% for the subordination. In the case of cortisol decreased it by 10 % of the dominant and increased with 15% for the subordination. Testosterone is the hormone that affects the body to instinct, risk-taking and social status thinking, while cortisol causes a negative stress on your body. Amy Cuddy draws the conclusion of the experiments that you yourself can affect their behavior even by adopting a fake power dominant condition as short as in a 2-minute before an important event such as a job interview or a public talk and through this influence the hormonal balance in the positive direction to be able to perform at the top.

So has research established the key in that which for example make a speek to convey a body language that reinforces and clarifies the verbal message you wish to convey. But also to read of his audience's reactions that feedback on to the message passed through. As noted in the previous chapter on intuition, it is often via body language we know of possible dissonance in it presented verbal expression. Amy Caddy's research also shows the important aspect that we ourselves may be affected by our own body language and that we can evolve through to take the requested position of power by affirmation in the face of important presentations

During the later years has it in the TV media stepped up various experts who have gone under the names horse whisper, dog or cat psychologists which are interpreter of the respective animal body language. It's striking how a horse whisper through their body language and behavior after just 5-10 minutes contact can have a completely unruly horse, which has not been able to be managed by its owner, to the quiet trot around and be controlled with easy care. Humans is also in high degree of how we are treated via body language. Research has shown that when we encounter a new alien man, so has our intuition and interpretation of body language on a few seconds created us a perception of the person-even properties that affect our relationship with the person of the future. Dress and appearance plays a major role in this context. In professions such as psychiatric aide and police playing the big role how it responds to clients with their body language and psychology, which as in horse whisper case can calm down an emergency situation or in the wrong body language at worst vice versa escalate behavior. A telling example is a management course in rational dialogue in which I participated, where they trained to negotiate and exercise was recorded on video for review afterwards. For two of the participants tracked the conversation gradually away, then their respective body languages triggered the other part to such attacks that the participants gone flamed at each other. Despite that it was a training exercise were affected people's continuation of the relationship in their normal life.

Body language dictionary

Body language is to their natural by various influences such as cultural impact and individual characteristics, but also of universal human expression. It is a lot of literature on how body language must be interpreted in detailed, but in this book is given only a few examples of body language which can be said to be universal. This follows a number of definitions of body language in literature.

• Eyes: Pupillary, range of eye movement.

• Posture: straight back, bend back, crossed the arms, approach, alienation, etc.

• Facial expressions: facial expressions, miner, Micro expression, Macro expression, etc.

• Voice: Pitch, melody, tempo, volume, fullness.

• Gestures: How we used, arms, legs, head movements to give signals.

The eyes are one of the important non- verbal signals where we usually have from childhood ability to read people's facial expressions. We can often at distances feel to have eye contact with a person, without to be able to see details of person's eyes. Pupil size is a marker unknowingly mirrors if we feel commitment and appreciation when they dilate. On the other hand, reflects the dissatisfaction or aggression when they draw up themselves if not surrounding bright light affect. A dithering worried look or gratuitous flashing can indicate that any lies, but it depends on the context if we shall be able to determine that there is no nervousness or eye problems behind.

Eye movement occurs not only when we use our eyes to follow a visual stimuli, without eyes tubes themselves also when we think of different things and also in a certain sleep called REM (Rapid Eye Movement). Eye movements linked to how we are going to have in brain research called Lateral Eye Movement. Within psychology school NLP (Neuro Linguistic Programming) so have Richard Bandler and John Grinder did research on how eye movements occurs when we are thinking of different things and created a model called the EAC (Eye Accessing Cues) in which it gives forms of range of eye movements. According to the model when we thinking about developing a memory image from the brain you move your eyes to the left. When you are constructing a new image so goes the eyes go to the right. A distinction is also looking up when it comes to a picture or straight to the side when it comes to a sound. Down the right for a physical sensation/feeling or finally down to the left when implementing an internal dialogue. When it comes to be able to expose a liar, so indicates a glance upwards to the right that you construct something new can be a lie. A look down to the left indicates that you think through something for yourself or a logical reasoning. Recent research has challenged the EAC model, but many argue that the model is practical useable.

Posture: The first man looks when it meets a human being is how the General posture looks. The first to describe the different body postures in his book Principles of Psychology, 1890, Ref. 6.4 was the American physiologist and Harvard Professor of psychology William James who studied human different postures and identified four different basic types and their psychological interpretation.

• Open, trust: an upright straight posture that gives a dominant and proud expression and showing on shelf condition.

• Crouching: a crouched stance indicating disappointment, resignation and may be the expression of a depression.

• Approach: A leaning forward posture indicating interest and a warm personality.

• Estranged: Opposite to the approach of shyness or a bored person with chilly stance.

William James pointed out in his research that there is a mutual depended between feelings and its expression in posture, but also the reverse that posture can affect the emotional state.

In the animal world as for e.g. monkeys so characterize the body language which rang a male monkey are within the Pack. Alpha male has a dominant performance by showing themselves big and powerful with broad brisket and even that hammer out of his chest. While a male in lower rank shows up resigned and itch alpha male on the back. The same behavior can be tracked in the contact between the human, where a power man often given special treatment and showing dominance in body language. As was mentioned earlier as showing Amy Caddy's research that we ourselves are affected by our own posture, which indicates that we should exercise at a more dominant image in the posture of that sounded to affect the surroundings on important issues and thus affect their confidence.

Already when you greet a new person by handshake, it can sometimes feel like a certain power struggle emerged as dominant unnecessarily hard handshakes can mark some kind of irritation between the parties. Even if the person turns the Palm down can it be a dominant marker while his hand in a normal vertical position indicates an interest in receiving. How to hold your arms can also indicate various feelings in an calls, such as to stand or sit with your arms crossed in front of him can be a marker of rejection or disinterest.

Facial expression: Facial expressions play a large role in how we experience the message and create contact in a conversation. As described earlier in the chapter so there are about 100 different facial expressions in FACS that we use on a regular call, but also humming, nodding, raised eyebrows or Micro expressions mark that people view the message and interact in the call.

Voice: How we use the voice plays also a great role and affects how we perceive the message at the verbal communication. When it comes to speakers, it is important to have a calm deep voice which is something melodious and not too monotonous. By varying the pitch and tempo can accentuate the bidding as it wants to convey. Language often reveals clearly from the background a new acquaintance comes from, where the dialect and slang language is clear you. In situations where you want to disclose any liar, so one should notice the voice shifts that can potentially detect misleading claims.

Gestures: People of all cultures use gestures in different contexts but here issued a warning in which meaning can vary a lot between different countries. When we thanks "Yes" through to nod, so will that interpreted the gesture as a "no" in Bulgaria, Turkey or Iran. A spontaneous gesture which is general is when a footballer or Boxer extending both arms in a gesture victory after a goal or a knock out. However, in a situation of war or police action to shows up hands that it gives up itself and consigns themselves to over power and shows that we do not have any weapons in their hands. Gestures to show "the finger" is an old insulting gesture in which the middle finger is said to symbolize a phallic symbol. But even the "V" sign taken from Churchill during World War II as a symbol of peace or profit, can be interpreted differently depending on if the back in or outside are turned towards the Viewer. In England, the Palm will be shown to the outside world if it is not to be interpreted as "fuck You".

As I said, so please refer to the bibliography if you want to immerse yourselves further in body language's many details.

This chapter on body language has shown how we unconsciously in "The Unconscious Zone" is affected by all the nuances expressed in body language such as facial expression, body posture, range of eye movement, voice and gesture. When we intuitively perceive a dissonances between verbal and non-verbal communication, become we often leery and vigilant against any lies. Mirror-neurons in our brain that reflects acts, intensions and emotions in people we consider, can be said to be behind man's unique capacity for compassion. We adjust us also often at the call after the other person's body language and tempo to show consensus and "we-feeling". A lesson learned from the researcher Amy Cuddy is to try to influence our own body language especially in important situations such as job interview or as speakers (even by that fake) through to affirmer a more dominant body language and thereby affect the hormonal balance in the body to be in top of the situation.

Chapter 7 Biofeedback

Conscious influence of the unconscious

The heading of this chapter point out available methods for affect many of the unconscious automated processes that regulate body functions via the autonomic nervous system. The autonomic nervous system consists of two parts called the sympathetic and the parasympathetic nervous system. The sympathetic nervous system affects the majority of the body's internal organ and activated when the body's forces mobilized as in stress situations or when you feel fear and enable stress hormones such as adrenaline and noradrenaline. These reactions make the body ready for escape or fight through, among other things increased heart rate, more blood to the muscles, increased blood pressure and digestion in save mode. Normally regulates the sympatric nervous system, among other things blood pressure and body temperature. The parasympathetic nervous system is most active at rest and calm situations to, among other things build up the body's reserve stock and immune system. The parasympathetic nervous system can be said to have opposite effect on the body than the sympathetic nervous system, which means a recovery of body power. In addition, a build-up of body reserves by, among other things heart rate reducer, blood pressure sinks, saliva production increaser, digestion and bowel movements increases and the natural emptying of bowel and urine is activated.

Under normal circumstances we do not consciously at all these nerve signals and hormone fluctuations that regulate the internal organ contained in "The Unconscious Zone". But it has been for millennia in the yoga traditions, meditation schools and with pranayama (breathing exercises) has been able to create conscious control of many of the autonomic nervous system functions as breathing, the heartbeat and body temperature. It has even been able to lower the metabolism and heart rhythm to a closest to the dazes State. In modern times, the Western medical research introduced methods that with electronic measurement instruments visualize different activities in the body with the help of sensors that measure such as heart rhythm and then presents this information visually or audial. Man has coined the term biofeedback for these methods from the word bios which interpreted life and feedback that means feedback. Biofeedback method is based on making the client aware of the body function you want to affect, and by the feedback from the measured variable is able to control its activity by the mind.

In connection with the rapid development of electronic measuring instruments during the 1950-1960's, so grew an intense research activity around the measurement of, among other things the electrical muscle signals (EMG) and the brain's internal electrical signals through EEG equipment. One of these pioneers was the American researcher Barbara Brown (1921-1999) originally had a doctorate in Pharmacology but then focused itself on psychic research and physiologic appeared as professor among others at the University of California. Barbara Brown was with and organized great Conference for feedback in Santa Monica United States 1969, where many of the leading scientists participated. The Conference resulted in the formation of organization The Biofeedback Research with Barbara Brown as the first President. Barbara suggested the new designation biofeedback for the new research area, which previously flourished under different name Muscle feedback, EEG feedback, Control of autonomic function accommodation. Barbara Brown became they who brought out the biofeedback research out to the general audience and published a number of high profile publications and books about research results and its possibilities. Two of her books "New Mind, New Body" (Harper & Raw, 1974) and "Stress and the art of biofeedback" (Harper & Raw, 1977) touched on research on brain electrical activities with the help of EEG measurements. Where a recognized experiment could control an electric train with Alpha waves captured from an experimental subject's brain. Stance against directly measuring brain activity via the EEG for feedback control has come to be called neurofeedback.

In her book "The hidden power", 1982, (see ref. 7.1) describes Barbara Brown how method biofeedback applied in two different types of experiments. Where to in case 1 deals with the disorder Raynaud's syndrome, a disease in which the hand's blood vessels constrict due to over activity in the sympatric nervous system and on the other hand, case 2 where volunteers can affect a specific muscle cells with desire. In case 1 with Raynaud's syndrome are often the hand cold and blue colored with pain due to poor blood circulation. Biofeedback is done by connecting biofeedback equipment that continuously measures the temperature of the hand and blood flow and present these metrics visually or audial. The exercise begins with that the patient gets background information about the condition and ground for the disease. The patient receives instructions on how she can use her psyche for to achieve a temperature increase in the hand through visualization, autosuggestion, or relaxation techniques. After a few training sessions, the patient learns to control the hand. When you ask the patient how they are doing to control the hand's temperature, they cannot describe how to do this or say that they put themselves in a different state of mind.

This is a clear demonstration of the active and unconscious learning in the same way as learning to ride a bike. Method has several torques in the mind where a visual idea of the measured temperature shall be interpreted/valued and then compiled with the sensation of heat or cold. The conceptual information (instructions, background information) and the biological information must be translated into just the sort of nervous activity that can be combined with certain mechanisms in mind and brain. The whole process takes place in the unconscious; it is the unconscious that controls the body and get it to perform precisely the action that the patient concerned with to raise the temperature in his hand. In large seen the same process occur most often at biofeedback learning to control internal body functions.

In experiment 2, is demonstrated the ability to mentally control the individual cells in the muscles. The electrical activity in the muscle cell can easily be measured with a sensor on the skin above the chosen muscle. With the help of amplifiers and an oscilloscope, the electrical signal to the muscle is visualized to the subject. When the average person get this information on muscle cell's work to teach them to control the muscle and make it surprisingly quickly. This is so much more surprising when you realize that every muscular and electric potential represents activity in a single motor neuron, i.e. each motor unit control the race a single motor neuron of spinal cord. Learning can take place in such a way that the person may select out a stimuli as to its form, size and accompanying audio signal can be detected on the oscilloscopes screen. The person is asked to guide its presence "on something mentally way". This is typically all information or instruction person get, but within a few minutes has he learned to check the measured quantity. Average people can also learn to check a dozen or more motor units individually or in group. Although it is astonishing that an individual on appeal can teach itself this so fast, is it than more surprising that a person learns to control cells without having anyone info on what is shown on the oscilloscopes screen. Once you have learned to control a body function the biofeedback equipment is no longer needed, which trained in the control function in the brain and can perform without external stimulus.

This ability to control the muscles used for example for prostheses for people who have lost an arm , and where we have been able to create a new artificial motorized arm that can be controlled in similar natural movements for the regular arm. This is done with measure sense with sensors on the skin of these motor nerves. When I did my diploma thesis at the Department of medical electronics at Chalmers Technical University in 1978, the Department was researched with specialized electronics which measured EMG signals and filtered out appropriate EMG signals for control of motors in a prosthetic arm.

In recent years, the development of biofeedback meant that a large number of sensors and electronic measuring equipment has been developed, where especially the fast computer development led to the sophisticated opportunities to present the measured biological measures to facilitate the client's perception and understanding. The following list presents a number of devices and sensors which are used both for medical diagnoses of e.g. hart disease, research purposes, lie detectors, measurement of sports men's health/fitness facilities and for biofeedback treatment of various diseases including the treatment of stress.

• Electromyography (EMG): EMG using surface electrodes on the skin above a muscle to measure muscle action potential from underlying skeleton muscles that initiates muscle contraction. The signals are weak in micro Volts area and noisy and treated with amplifier and filtering to be useful.

• Feedback thermometer: measuring skin temperature with a thermistor as a sensor and can measure temperature with large accuracy (1/100 degree C). Normally connect the sensor to a finger or a toe and the client gets a visual or audio based indication as temperature increases or decrease.

• Elektrodermografi (EDG): measures the skin's electrical conductance and skin potential with electrodes on the client's hand or wrist. Measurement of skin resistance indicates excitement, anxiety and cognitive activity, then skin resistance reduces when you sweat. These sensors are used for a long time in the context of lie detectors.

• Electroencephalography (EEG): EEG measures the electric activity in the cerebral cortex through electrodes placed on the scalp. EEG use precious metal electrodes and measure the voltage between two electrodes on the scalp, but usually has a hat with a larger number of electrodes that can view the activity in different parts of the cerebral cortex.

• Electrocardiogram (ECG): ECG typically use electrodes placed on the torso, which records the electrical activity of the heart and heart rate checks and any disease in the heart.

• Photoplethysmograf (PPG): PPG measure blood flow with a sensor attached to the fingers or the temporal that measure flow with an infrared light source that transmitted through or reflected from tissue.

• Pneumograf: consists of a flexible sensor band with string strain sensor which is placed around the chest or abdomen to measure breathing rate.

• Capnometer measures the pressure of the carbon dioxide in exhaled air through a plastic tube placed in the nostril. Used for the control of breathing quality.

• Rhevencephalograf (REG): REG measuring brain blood flow at bio-feedback. The electrodes attached to the head and measure connectivity of tissue between the electrodes.

• Hemoecephlograf (HEG): measures the differences in infrared light reflected from the scalp and show the relative amount of oxygenated blood and non-oxygenated blood in the brain.

• Functional magnetic resonance imaging (fMRI): the method is a further development of magnetic resonance imaging (MRI), but where you can view the difference in blood flow in various parts of brain by color coding of the tomography picture in real time. To generate an image required exposure about 2 seconds.

• Diffusion tensor imaging (DTI): the method maps the brain's neural networks by following diffusion of water molecules in myelin tissue of neuronal axons (outputs).

• Magnetoencephalography (MEG): Equipment that directly measures the magnetic field outside the scalp. When the signals from cerebral synapses are weak must the equipment be used in MEG magnetically shielded room. Gives good time resolution but require approximately 50000 neurons at the same time is active for a good signal quality.

• Transcranial Magnetic stimulation (TMS): Equipment with directed magnetic field for the influence of synapse function.

• Transcranial Direct Current Stimulation (TDCS): Equipment for injecting a weak direct current for the influence of synapse function.

In the continuation of this book will a number of applications in the following areas to be described as an example of the rapid development of biofeedback methods in the last few decades.

- Neuro-feedback

- Lie detectors

- Expert training of brain to operate in "the zone"

- Computer control for disabled people

- Game controlled by EEC signals

Neuro-feedback

In biofeedback research in recent decade has been an explosive development in the area which are referred to as neurofeedback. The new sophisticated equipment for EEG and fMRI measurement has created entirely new opportunities to identify the brain's various areas and measure was different cognitive and motor activities are carried out and in real time, view the dynamic process that goes on in the brain.

At measurement of EEG signals from the client it is possible to note a number of characteristic waveforms in the signals that reflect the subject's consciousness. In table 7.1 shows a compilation and classifying of the brain rhythm signals that you can get at the EEG measurement depends on the client's State of consciousness

Frequency interval	Associated with:	EEG
> 40 Hz Gammawaves	Higer mental skill as problem solving, fear and alertness.	
13–39 Hz Betawaves	Active nervous thoughts, active concentration, elated.	
7–13 Hz Alfawaves	Alert relaxation, prelimary sleep, dazed, REM-sleep och dreaming.	
4–7 Hz Thetawaves	Deep meditation, sleep.	
< 4 Hz Deltawaves	Deep, dreamless sleep.	

Table 7.1 EEG wave form (Källa: wikipedia.org/wiki/Elektroencefalografi).

The lower frequencies in the delta (< 4 Hz) and theta waves (4-7 Hz) is characterized by deep sleep or deep meditation and the client is not awake consciousness. Most interesting is the alpha waves (7-13 Hz) that characterize a person with eyes closed is mentally relaxed yet awake, but also occurs in the so-called REM sleep characterized by rapid eye movements with closed eyes. If the person opens the eyes or distracted by something weakens the alpha waves and instead activates the brain and the faster beta waves (13-40 Hz) becomes dominant. Alpha waves' showing in what degree the brain is itself in a state of relaxed attention that characterizes an open and creative state of consciousness in which contact with the emotions and the subconscious can give new impression. Investigation of, for example yogis during meditation show that the presence of alpha waves increase. At deep meditation in the advanced stages of yogis is an increased presence of theta waves (4-7 Hz). Measurement of EEG signals showing that the level of Alpha waves can be different in the left and right brain. The left hemisphere which handle verbal, analytical and logical thinking while the right hemisphere manage emotional, musical and spatial perception leads to left hemisphere thinks in words and concepts while right thinking in pictures, feeling and sensations. Typically shifts the balance of alpha waves spontaneously between right and left hemisphere, depending on the activity that you do.

During the early research with help of EEG measurement during 1950-1960 performed by, among other things Professor of psychology, Joe Kamiya at the University of Chicago was made in conjunction with sleep research experiment in which the client would learn to recognize when alpha waves produced. The experiment was performed so that during the time the EEG measurement was carried out so called the investigator in a clock at various random times in which case the client would answer (A) and (B) if he thought that Alpha or Beta waves were produced. The investigator gave direct feedback about the answer was with EEG registration. At the first day's experiments so got only 50% correct answers which are purely random. During the second day increased the outcome right answer to 60% and on day three to 80%. During day four correct answers increased to 85% and continued efforts with this client led to almost 100% correct answers were obtained. The trials showed that the feedback could teach the client to recognize when alpha waves produced. Results in other subjects varied, and to see if direct feedback could increase learning ability was a biofeedback equipment development witch measured the Alpha presence in EEG signals and gave an audio tone when Alpha waves appeared. With this equipment in which the client himself got directly feedback at the presence of the alpha waves as increased learning ability and some clients were able to generate alpha waves on command from the investigator and also move the dominant Alpha frequencies 1 Hz. When test results published with an article in the publication "Psychology Today", 1968 was a large impact and created a boom in the United States for EEG biofeedback equipment for training of alpha waves. It is thought that the training of alpha waves would with-keep a quick way to get new meditative state of consciousness, but this fashion trend slowed down pretty quickly.

Professor emeritus Barry Sterman at the University of California, Los Angeles, who worked on sleep research during the 1960's, discovered in 1965 by research with cats a new type of EEG waves that came to be called SMR (sensorimotor rhythm) with rhythmic waves in the frequency range 12-15 Hz. EEG electrodes were placed over the parts of the cortex that deal with the body's movements and that is called motor cortex. At attempts were electrodes implanted in the cats ' brains in order to get so undisturbed and localized EEG registrations as possible. The trials were conducted with 30 cats as before the trials got very little food for to be motivated for rewards in the form of bread and milk. At attempts were placed the cat in a Chamber with a lever that gave the bread and milk in a bowl each time the cat pressed the lever. Then introduced a moment to when the cat heard a tone had he no food at the operation of the lever, but when the tone stop they worked the lever again. The researchers noted that the cats came in a unique state of mind, where they were themselves quite still but on edge which is similar to the condition the cats take on the hunt for mice or birds. This condition of EEG registrations with signals in the frequency range 12-15 Hz, which was localized from electrodes placed in cerebral motor cortex. The trials were developed further by the lever was taken away and the cat got food when the self-produced SMR waves for half a second. After training the cats could get his reward that they themselves could produce SMR waves with his will. These unique results are reported in 1967 in the medical journal "Brain Research" (see ref. 7.2).

Sterman was contacted by the space agency NASA about the astronauts and workers who handled the rocket fuel (monometylhydrazin, MMH) could get hallucinations and severe epileptic seizures when handling rocket fuel. Sterman used 50 cats for new trials, of which 10 had been included in the earlier SMR training. When the cats were injected with rocket fuel so they ended up in a chaotic State and after an hour got the strong epileptic seizures. The ten cats that concluded in the previous SMR training were only those who escaped the attacks for any reason. Sterman realized that the 10 cats that have undergone SMR training had strengthened its brain, which had raised the threshold in brain cells that end up in epileptic seizures. Sterman started research on patients who suffered from epilepsy to see if he could get the same effect with reduction of the assault. A feedback out-armor that via a green light shone at the SMR waves and a red light on SMR did not occur was applied to the patient. The patient was trained to keep the green light stays on and the red led is off. The result was overwhelming when the epileptic attacks decreased by 65%. The results were published in the medical journal Epilepsia, 1978, "Effects of central cortical EEG feedback training on incidence of poorly controlled seizures" (see ref. 7.3). Today, it is an established method of treating epilepsy patients.

A different scientist Professor emeritus Joel Luber at University of Tennessee as studied diseases ADD/ADHD with, among other things overactive children read the Sterman reports on treatment of epilepsy and realized that similar reactions of motor cortex of hyperactive children. Luber worked together with Sterman during a year and studied effect of SMR on children with ADHD diagnosis. The children were trained with SMR feedback until their symptoms subsided and revealed that it was a successful method for the treatment of ADHD. The method used today for treatment of ADHD.

The area with the EEG operated neurofeedback has been developed with the new method to deal with the EEG signals with different mathematical analysis such as Fourier analysis, which is called qEEG, which provided new opportunities for presentation of EEG results. Among other things can you view a number of images which are called "brain maps" where we divided the EEG signal frequency content so that each image shows a color coded surface with qEEG signal amplitude over cortex surface for a given frequency band, for example. 12-15 Hz, this means that you can compare some standardized EEG signals stored in databases for comparison in the treatment of diseases such as epilepsy. EEG guided neurofeedback has applications in many areas such as substance abuse, migraine, depression, autism, epilepsy and stroke treatment.

Through the new fast computers and effectiveness of computer algorithms in the neurofeedback field during the 2000 's have new magnetic resonance equipment (fMRI) taken up which shows brain's varying blood flows as in real time can be presented to the client. You can dynamically show snapshots of the brain, where areas with high blood circulation can color coded and thereby to the difference from EEG registration show blood flow in 3D with higher resolution in real time. One of the researchers behind the new functional magnetic resonance equipment with real-time presentation is Dr. Christopher deCharms as the research team have been with and developed the new partly patented technology rt-fMRI (real time functional magnetic resonance tomography). One of the functions that it conducted research in is the treatment of patients with chronic pain, in which the usual treatments with medicines and acupuncture has shown poor results with pain relief. In a study conducted at Stanford University under the heading "Control over brain accusation and pain learned by using real-time functional MRI" reported in the Proceedings of the National Academy of Science of the United States in 2005, (see ref. 7.4), so set to two basic questions that you want to highlight with the study.

• Can a person learn through feedback to verify a designated part of the brain that is involved in pain experiences called anterior cingulate cortex (rACC).

• Can the person have an impact in terms of reducing pain experiences in both a group of healthy individuals and in a group of patients with long run chronic pain.

The experiments started with a group of 8 healthy persons were examined in an rt-fMRI equipment. To generate a pain perception so joined a computer-controlled device that was applied on the arm and that when it gave a heat pulse on the skin. The subject was given grade level of pain on a scale from 0 = no pain, to 10 = the worst possible pain. They scanned a subject's brain during activation of pain and saw a strong reaction in anterior cingulate cortex (rACC). They performed test in which asked volunteers to affect brain activity when it got featured an animated flame whose intensity varied with the measured blood flow to the painful area, via a couple of Computer controlled glasses. The results showed that the subject could affect blood flow through feedback and reduce pain. The experiment showed that the first and second questions could be answered with a Yes. The experiment continued with 8 patients who suffered from chronic pain. The experiment was carried out in the same way as with the healthy group, but now patients were instructed to affect their own chronic pain. At evaluation of the results there was got an reduction of pain with 64%. Further studies are under way in various areas such as treatment of depression, stroke, ADHD and post-traumatic stress.

The Method with rt-fMRI has a great future potential for the treatment of patients, for example with more severe chronic pain conditions, then the equipment requires a large local, trained personnel and are expensive investments. There is a potential to build program modules which can be adapted individually for each patient, where you can select how the presentation of feedback information to be carried out and various algorithms for the analysis of various medical conditions. In a future would a patient be able to get a form before treatment where you can choose how the feedback information will be displayed e.g. a variable flame, diverse bars with various colors or varying tones and where the processor has access to the library of algorithms for various medical conditions for proper data collection and presentation.

Lie detectors

Lie detectors in the form of polygraphs has during long time used in the United States by the Federal police, the FBI and CIA during interrogations in order to be able to expose any lies during interrogations. The method itself has been called into question, but biofeedback equipment has gradually been refined from early only EDG electrodes for the measurement of skin conductance to that in today's "polygraphs" have at least 4 to 5 different measurement electrodes EDG, measuring respiratory rate ECG or blood pressure and sometimes motion detector from foot/leg. The measurements are displayed on a computer screen in the form of 4 curves that continuously shows the suspect's reactions. Questions are marked with their time on screen in order to be able to relate to each response. At polygraph testing used different query techniques to be able to determine if and when the suspect lies. The most widely used technique in testing of suspected criminal cases is the CQT (control question test) with Yes or No asked questions, where comparisons of polygraph outcomes relevant questions about the crime and control questions. The relevant issues are of type

"Shot you person NN" while control questions are more general and often if previous phenomena such as "have you ever revealed someone who trusted on you". The tests are based on the assumption that a person who speaks truth react most in control questions that are asked on their previous life while the relevant issues they know that they are not interested in. While the adoption of a guilty person is that he reacts more strongly on the relevant questions than control subjects. The interrogator, who is specially trained polygraph interpretation, begins the hearing by asking questions to see how the response looks during normal conversation before he goes in with direct questions about the suspected were interference in the investigated crime. In the literature indicated that the modern polygraphs with the appropriate trained interpreters can have a probability of up to 90 % to identify future lies in irrigates.

As described with examples in the chapter body language, so going on research projects in which it examines new areas for the detection of lies that computer analysis of facial Micro expressions, examination with fMRI of cerebral blood flow by lies and something that has been called "brain fingerprint" where man with EEG registration can measure a special pulse in wave pattern which is called P300. This alert indicates that if a query generates this pulse subconsciously when you access a stored memory out of the brain. The name "brain fingerprint" shall refer to the corresponding finger prints which are used as evidence in the crime investigations. Researcher Dr. Lawrence Farwell has developed patented computer controlled equipment for detection of "brain fingerprint" signals that have been used in research for, among other things CIA and FBI associated with Harward Medical School. In several rapports among others: Farwell LA, Richardson DC., Richardson GM, 2008, "Brain fingerprinting field studies comparing P300_MERMER and P300 brainwave responses in the detection of concealed information", Cognitive Neurodynamics, (see ref. 7.5), sets out for the patented method.

The clients which are examined are provided with an electrode band around the head and with a deal that passes right through the scalp from nape to forehead. The latter electrode band have three electrodes, on the other hand, in the middle of the scalp and one in front lobe and one in neck lobe of the scalp. The band around the head has two electrodes, one on each side of the forehead above the eyes. A reference electrode is connected by the ear. From the headband are the electrodes connected to an EEG device that records EEG signals. Method is based on a unique signal called the P300 witch is generated about 300 milliseconds after the client has seen a sentence or a picture of something that is stored in his brain, while this signal fails if it is unknown to him.

Lawrence Farwell has in cooperation with the CIA and the FBI conducted a number of experiments in which they have been able to identify for example FBI agents through to view conditions or secret codes that only these agents know to. At trial with agents each randomly selected subjects to have the method in about 200 trials demonstrated 100 % correct identification of the agents as part of the efforts. The method is considered to be able to identify terrorists or bomb makers, to see on the response at the display of data that only someone in a terrorist cell is aware of. Procedure in the event of a "brain fingerprint" survey goes to so that the client provided with headband with electrodes connected to a computer based EEG equipment for registration. In front of the client is a monitor placed where the information (pictures, sounds, words or phrases) will be shown in about 300 ms (milliseconds) controlled by a computer program and at the same time collect the EEG data during 2 seconds. Then presented new information's and with new EEG recording etc. until sufficient probability for analysis of data can occur. In order to ensure that the measurements are calibrated are the information divided into three categories with 15% target data, 70% irrelevant data and 15 % probe data. Target is generic information known by the person who shall serve as reference in EEG signal, while the largest part data is 70% irrelevant information serves as feedback of non-notable info and works as a reference while the probe data is the relevant information that only the perpetrator knows if it committed the crime. The signals are processed with computer algorithms known as P300 MERMER to filter out the final signal on that data is stored or not stored in memory.

The interesting thing with this method is that it has been used by American court where there in a case with a prisoner of Mr. Harrington who was sentenced in 1978 to life imprisonment of the "Supreme Court of the State of Iowa" for the murder of a police officer Mr. John Schweer which was committed in 1977. Harrington, who was 17 years old at the time, was convicted without having confessed the murder and with weak evidence with only a witness who at that time was 16 age. The case came to light in 2000 when Harrington asked rising in goal and in connection with this was called Dr. Farwell to do a test with the method "brain fingerprint" (see figure 7.2). The test showed that Harrington did not have any "hits" on things that had to do with the crime, but on the other hand, when it was his alibi. After the case was taken up again 2003 after the Harrington spent more than 25 years in prison, he was released from prison and got a large indemnity paid.

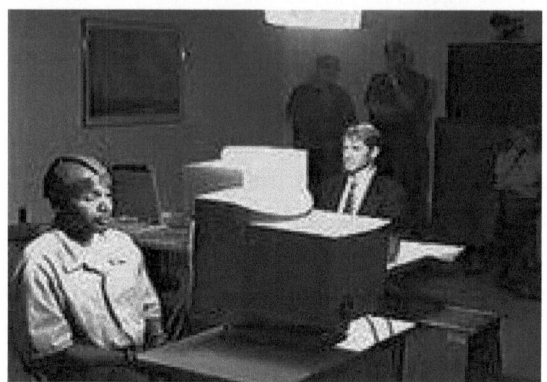

Fig. 7.2 Dr. Lawrence Farwell conducts a Brain Fingerprinting test on Terry Harrington.
(Källa: http://en.wikipedia.org/wiki/Brain_fingerprinting)

"Brain fingerprint" was performed also on serial killer James B Ginder. Dr. Farwell was approached by Sheriff Robert Dawson to perform a test to see if there was information that matched the details of the murder of Julie Helton. The test turned to information if the murder was in memory and Ginder he decided himself to admit the murder when he otherwise surely condemned to death penalty. Ginder was sentenced to life in prison without the possibility of grace. He later admitted murdering three more women.

Expert training of brain for effect in "the zone"

A new area of application for EEG measurement with neurofeedback is examination of experts carried out a study of three archers in the U.S. Olympic national team, four Professional golfer in PGA tour and thirteen snipers that served as professional trainers of rifle snipers. The study is reported in a report: "Accelerating Training using interactive neuro educational technologies: Applications to archery, golf and rifle marksmanship", Chris Berka, Adrianne Behneman, Natalie Kintz, Robin Johnson and Gitsy Raphael, The International Journal of sport & society (see ref. 7.6).

The intension of the study was to identify how EEG brainwave from a number of experts looked like when they were in the "zone" i.e. the crucial State of concentration before the firing of an arrow, when hitting a golf ball or trigger rifles. They were interested by what that separates a beginner and a possible Olympic champion when it comes to brain function in the blink of an eye, for example when you are aiming and releasing the arrow for an Archer. The study showed part of a general pattern in EEG signals to all the experts, but also that there were minor differences between the three disciplines. In this representation there are sets out only the results for the archers. The result for the intrepid Archer was three seconds ahead of the release of arrow to increase gradually the percentage of Alpha waves (8-12 Hz) and theta waves (3-7 Hz) up to the launching moment in all six measured EEG channels.

The study went on to see if it can shorten the learning curve for beginners in the respective areas, by using biofeedback equipment help the adept to come into the same mental state "zone" as the advanced practitioner has in sight and shooting time (Peak performance). The leader of the study Chris Berker who is CEO of the company ABM (Advanced Brain Monitoring) and working with the company's research and development of EEG based devices for feedback, initiated the start of developing a feedback equipment of that train beginners which came to be called APPT (Adaptive Peak Performance Trainer). Input to the design was the experts ' brain waves when they were in the "zone" (Peak Performance). It filtered EEG waves as experts and set up criteria when alpha waves reached over two limits of 5% and 10%. The beginners in archery were measured EEG signals with a headband and feedback was provided with two small vibrators mounted on adept shirt collar. When the vibrator a hushed had it reached the first boundary for Alpha waves at 5 % and when both silenced had reached "the zone" for firing 10% alpha waves. The results showed that the normal learning curve to become expert in this case where archery could be reduced by 240%. As we saw by research on expertise in chapter 5 to talk to about magnitude 10000 hours of practice to become a professional musician in the world, indicating that with the help of APPT equipment so should they in a future to decrease training time for a beginner drastically and even for experienced practitioners can expert exercise be an effective help in improving performance. These devices have great potential as training facilities for sport and have even been tried in the United States armed forces for training by snipers.

Computer control for people with disabilities

In neurofeedback research regarding EEG signals which means to computer controlled communication aid for hard disabled like for i.e. ALS patients, which gradually loses the ability to speak and to be able to move arms and legs. They have to design equipment that is controlled through mental functions in the brain. As an example, a piece of equipment called iBrain, which consists of a band around the head with a small box that measures the brain EEG signals which are transmitted wirelessly to a computer for analysis. The equipment is developed by the researcher Philip Low, who founded the company NeuroVigil and iBrain used since 2009 for measuring sleep problems, drug research on the brain, depression and Alzheimer's disease. Application of ALS patients are supposed to be able to identify the EEG signals in the brain's motor cortex , which for an ALS patient still generated, but the disease has destroyed neurons that shall enable the muscle activity. The computer program contains algorithm that identifies the EEG waves that are generated when you plan on touching the left or right arm and who can control a cursor on the computer screen. The computer system can then generate synthetic speech or writing according to which sentences are built up. Philip Low has worked with the two famous people Dr. Stephan Hawkins who is known for his work with black holes and "Big bang" in physics and Augie Nieto who built up a large company in the "life fitness" before he 2005 were affected by ALS. Dr. Hawkins affected by ALS in 25 years of age and gradually became paralyzed in muscles lost speech in 1985. Despite this can he today lead a TV program in channel Discovery Science about universe thanks through a computer equipment which through glasses with infrared light feel of muscle activity in the cheek and control point in a computer that generates synthetic speech. In the same way hit Augie Nieto of ALS in 2005 that gradually led to he today only can communicate with the movement of the toes that via a control ball can operate a computer with speech synthesis. Augie Nieto has together with his wife founded an organization, as collected in over 400 million dollars for research on ALS. Philip Low has examined the two patients with the help of iBrain equipment and map their EEG wave pattern in the motor cortex and been able to decode the signals that would normally turn right or left hand. Thus, one can control a cursor through mental activity on a computer and via speech synthesizer to express them, write text and click to pass up on the internet. When ALS progresses so maybe the last remnants of Hawkins and Nieto muscle activity disappear and then they would be able to be an option with iBrain control for communication and speech synthesis.

Game controlled by EEG signals

During later time have it brought out many Games at the entertainment market that use EEG signals via headband for to control the games. An early game on the market is "Mindball game" which was developed by the company Interactive Productline in Sweden which was introduced in 2003. The game is often used as the arcade games at exhibitions or science center and consists of a table on which two players sitting on opposite side of the table, with headbands connected to a computing device for evaluation of participants ' EEG waves. In the middle of the table is a spline between two endpoints that a ball can roll back and forth controlled by a mobile magnet under the table. The both gamers EEG alpha waves (8-12 Hz) and theta (4-8 Hz) are evaluated and on a monitor at the side of the table shows each attendee's alpha and theta signals chart. The participants shall put in a maximum of relaxed to able with closed eyes that provides a high level of

Alpha and theta waves in the EEG signals. The equipment is featured via the magnet ball against it that is at least relaxed. Research at Imperial College in London have shown that the exercise of the alpha and theta waves in the study of 100 students at the Royal College of music got better learning skills and passed the exam in the higher grade. The company has taken up an equipment called "Mindball Trainer" designed to improve relaxation ability and concentration of a person who on the corresponding way steering a ball on a smaller course. In this equipment can be set in 10 different levels in order to gradually be able to work out the alpha/theta waves to higher level. These devices marketed among other things to NASA for training of astronauts and to schools for improved learning.

To conclude this chapter on biofeedback, which demonstrated the future potential that are in computer-controlled equipment, to be an example of the ancient knowledge that through yoga and meditation can control the body's autonomic nervous system. At the beginning of the 20th century, so did the Belgian/French woman Alexandra David-Neel travel to India and Tibet as Explorer with interest for Buddhism and Tibetans philosophy and religious traditions. In 1924 made her a trip to Lhasa in Tibet which at that time was forbidden for Westerners to visit. Their experiences portrayed her in 1929 in her most famous book "Magic and Mystery in Tibet". She describes in the book how lamas who pulled himself back as hermits in caves in the mountain had through meditation practices check their body temperature so that they could sit out naked in the snow but not to freeze. Similar capabilities shall be presented by the Dutch world record-holder Wim Hof, which is an adventurer called for "ice man" for his ability to withstand the cold. According to the book Guinness World Record so have Wim Hof world record in to sit naked completely covered by ice cubes in 1 hour 52 minutes and 42 seconds. Hof indicates that through concentration and meditation so he can influence his autonomic nervous system by vagus nerve so that the thermostat in the body retains the normal body temperature and also affects the immune system. Hof has been giving out the book "Becoming the iceman ", 2011 and hold courses for interested in his meditation technique.

The autonomic nervous system, which is included in "The Unconscious Zone", as shown in this chapter are influenced both by consciously ancient practices like yoga and meditation, but now also via biofeedback with sophisticated electronic equipment and direct reading of the brain's electrical signals EEG. The fast computer development will generate future neurofeedback equipment as previously described in science fiction literature. In medicine play already biofeedback equipment a major role in the treatment of many diseases and neurological conditions such as epilepsy, ADHD, post-traumatic stress, autism, stroke, etc. It is also a great potential for accessibility for disabled persons.

Chapter 8 Hypnosis

Unconscious influences

In contrast to the previous chapter on the conscious action of the unconscious with biofeedback or with psychoanalysis methods, so are hypnosis methods that affect the psyche of a client in unconscious way. Hypnosis state is very similar to trance, where the normal knowledge level is affected. At first in this chapter follows a review of hypnosis history with emphasis on some important person's contribution to the hypnosis current position.

Trance state like hypnosis has been around so long as mankind evolved further from the stage of animals (Homo-Erectus). Even before the birth of Christ, there is evidence for those methods like hypnosis was used in various ancient cultures and mystery schools. Trance state has been used as a cure for various illnesses of many old cultures as in Hinduism in India, in ancient Egypt and Greece. It is used for example "Holy Temple" in Egypt, which is mentioned as dream temples, for over 4000 years ago in treatment of often psychological problems where treatment was given with meditation, fasting, various baths, dieter and adjudication by the patient in various trance states. Often included dream interpretation of priests who judged the treatment to be given.

Avicenna (Ibn Sina) (980-1037) was a psychologist and physician from Persia as 1027 published the book "The book of healing ", where he mentions the early forms of suggestions methods that can be interpreted as precursors to hypnosis. Avicenna was also a pioneer in Neuropsychiatry in which he described numerous neuropsychiatric problems as hallucination, insomnia, mania, nightmare, melancholy, dementia, epilepsy, paralysis, stroke, vertigo and tremor. Avicenna developed methods to treat emotional disorders and had a system that via the pulse read clients during patient call and know of any problem areas.

The Mesmerism

Franz Anton Mesmer (1734-1815) is considered to be one of the early pioneers of suggestions treatments historically mentioned laying the foundations for the modern hypnosis development. Messmer is behind the concept of "Animal magnetism", which was based on the passing of faith that there was a magnetic substance in the body to "animate" beings (those who breathe). Mesmer was of the opinion that if these magnetic gases were in imbalance in the body led to the illness occurred. Messmer was influenced by a Hungarian astronomer and Jesuit priest Maxmilian Hell (1720-1792) who was Director of the Observatory in Vienna. Hell was also interested of magnet therapy and worked as a healer using magnets that were placed on the skin of the patients. Mesmer was influenced as a young doctor and become a pupil of Hell.

In the beginning of his career used Mesmer a liquid that contained iron as the client had to drink before the body was treated with magnets on the different spots on the body. Patients reported feeling a mysterious power in the body that affects disease symptoms for several hours. Later realized Mesmer that there was no need of magnets for treatment but that it was "The Magnetizer" which affected patients directly. After a controversy with the failure of treatment of a blind girl 1777 so left he Vienna for to try to establish himself in Paris. The first years in Paris, he failed to get his theories of animal magnetism that is accepted by the medical establishment Royal Society of Medicine. But he managed to enlist a professor of medicine Charles d ' Eston as his pupil and collaborator. His methods became fashionable and made a success in the treatment of nervous problems within the aristocracy. 1779 wrote Mesmer in collaboration with d ' Eston an 88 page book "Memorie sur la decouvertr du magnetisme animal" in which he gave an account of their theories.

To start with treated Mesmer their patients individually as he sat near and in contact with the patient's knees and for longer periods of time focused areas of the abdominal region by hand printing and gazed intensely in their eyes. The response from patients was often with strong feelings and convulsions that were seen as part of the treatment. When the patient influx increased introduced Mesmer a method for to be able to be treated many patients at the same time by introducing a large thin "baquet" with metal rods jutting out of the lid. In the barrel low glass bottles with magnetized water stacked and in contact with moving bent iron bars on the top cover. Iron Rails were placed on different parts of patients ' bodies for treatment. Thus could a larger number of patients treated at a time and bring higher revenues by business. Mesmer as dressed in kaftans walked around with a "magnetic pole" and touched patients to reinforce effect of the treatment. Women who were in the majority among the patients were often attack with spastic seizures, rattling breath and gave loud cries. Many women with hysterical disorders and nervous young men from high society were treated in the business witch served Mesmer big money.

Mesmer's success was seen with harsh eyes of the rest of the medical society in Paris and King Louis XVI started a Commission of scientists who would examine the Mesmer's theories on a scientific way. The Commission included the chemist Antoine Lavoisier, the physicist Joseph-Ignae Guillotin, the astronomer Jean Sylvan Bailly and the American Ambassador Benjamin Franklin. The Commission made a number of experiments with, among other things Mesmer's Assistant Charles d ' Eston and came up to be someone "animal magnetism" did not exist and the method was based on sheer "fantasies". Mesmer was forced to leave Paris and his practice but the Government gave him a pension. There were opponents against the Commission's findings, which meant that only in terms of scientific results and do not take into account the results of the Mesmer's methods had given on patients ' recovery.

Mesmer's ideas about animal magnetism continued to be practiced by many followers who for example Marquis Puységur (1751-1825) which coined the concept "artificial somnambulism" after to have treated a patient who fell in a deep trance that resembled a deep sleep condition named somnambulism. Puységur got like Mesmer many patients and to be able to treat all magnetized he a tree that would be affected of patients for transfer of the magnetic force and the tree was called "Puységur 's tree". Mesmer's ideas were taken up in several countries as for example Germany, England and Switzerland and were called Mesmerism.

James Braid and hypnosis concept

In the further hypnosis development can include Charles Lafontaine (1803-1892) a Swiss living in Geneva who was Publisher of a journal called "Le magnétiseur" and which was a traveling "magnetizer" in Mesmer's spirit. At a demonstration of animal magnetism in Manchester England 1841 became the Scottish surgery James Braid (1795-1860) first skeptical to the demonstration. Lafontaine appeared as an artist with long black beard with a penetrating gaze and would put the subject in a State insensitive to pain. By giving the person electric shock with a battery and burn with a burning wax candles was demonstrated client's insensitivity to pain. Braid became interested and visited a demonstration six days later to reveal bluff, but at confrontation with the subject he realized that it was a genuine effect which affected the client. Braid began experimental era of hypnosis among his friends, his wife, and later also with patients. When Braid was, among other things specialist on eye diseases noted he that it was easiest to put people in a hypnotic state by the client was staring at a shiny object such as a coin, in front of their eyes and, depending on muscle effort around the eyes placed person in hypnotic state and often closes his eyes automatically. Braid charted by different experiment how the hypnotic state spoke, and in one of the experiments, he noted that a client in waking heard a ticking clock at 3 feet while in the hypnotic state as he heard the clock from 35 feet i.e. 12 times so far.

Braid found that there Mesmerism explained the hypnotic to estate with animal magnetism, magnetic gases or emphasis of "magnetizer" ability, so was the hypnotic state at the client's own psychological factors and client's concentration on one object. In start associated Braid hypnosis state as a form of sleep, but experiment turned instead to a focused attention was behind hypnosis. Braid coined the term "nervous sleep" and used the

189

term hypnosis as the first in the English linguistic realm from the Greek word hypnosis which means sleep. Braid tried to later introduce the term monoideism instead of Hypnosis State to emphasize the significance but failed, so that the term hypnosis became the predominant. James Braid has come to be seen as that which defined the word hypnosis and emphasized the psychological background to hypnosis state by creating a theoretical model based on psychology and induction with simple methods. He clarified the hypnotic state that for example catalepsy, immobility in muscle, and the ability to post hypnotic state, (suggestions carried out unconsciously by the client on the post hypnotic command after awakening). Braid thought that hypnosis could affect different parts of the brain to change a client's behavior and that it could affect many automatic body processes as for example heart rate and blood pressure during trance. Through his studies and experiments with hypnosis gave Braid scientific legitimacy to hypnosis as a clinical method for treatment of many psychological illnesses and he is considered to be one of the first to be called Hypnotherapist.

Braid used Hypnotherapy for the treatment of a number of medical conditions that stroke, paralyzing condition, chronic rheumatism, headache and sensory problems. In his book "Neurhypnology" which was published in 1843 describes Braid 25 different cases which he treated as a Hypnotherapist but also cases where hypnosis methods did not work. Braid thought that hypnosis only would be used by Professional staff in the medical context and not be used as esterified entertainment.

In the early 1800's, there was no access to chemical anesthetics for surgery operations until when ether was introduced in 1846 and chloroform 1847. In the American civil war and in British India was used with success hypnosis as analgesia to block pain and reduce bleeding by i.e. amputation. Doctor James Esdaile (1805-1859) carried out e.g. 345 major operations at a hospital in the city of Hooghly India with the help of hypnosis techniques that built on Mesmerism and reached 50% better results in terms of mortality (8%). These results probably depended on the great acceptance that existed in India for unorthodox methods and that the Esdaile had assistants who put patients in a deep hypnosis (called the Esdaile state) during a long induction, (sometimes a whole day) in order to reach the deepest hypnosis states.

Paris and Nancy school

During the latter part of the 1800's came two directions in the hypnosis which is often referred to as the Paris school and Nancy school. In Paris seemed to Jean-Martin Charot (1825-1893), who was a senior physician at the mental hospital Salpetriere and treated patients with hysteria and believed that only patients with predisposition for hysteria could be subject for hypnosis. Charot was also one of the first who investigated and classified different hypnosis deep and named the three levels Lethargy, Catalepsy and Somnambulism.

Nancy school with A A Liébeault (1823-1907) and Hippolyte Bernheim (1840-1919) argued, however, that hypnosis was a form of suggestion. Liébeault and Bernheim had a clinic together and treated 30000 patients during a 20-year period, with an emphasis on easy hypnosis and verbal suggestion technics where the patient was conscious of the treatment after the awakening. Their success with treatments meant that many doctors came to study their methods of which Sigmund Freud was one.

Freud translated, among other things Bernheims book on hypnosis "The la Suggestion" to German and practiced during a period of hypnosis as a psychotherapy method. Freud changed his approach to hypnosis when he with his colleague Joseph Breuer studied the historical case of Bertha Pappenheim named as Anna O which showed a number of hysterical symptoms would probably depends of her strict parents during her childhood . She could during the treatment of the family doctor Breuer go in self-hypnosis and were treated over a two-year period for its alternating symptoms such as hallucination, symptoms of paralysis in the face, arms and legs, at times lost speech, etc. During the treatments, she told about childhood experiences drawn from fairy tales and when her father died after a year's illness was she in a major crisis. During the ongoing treatment with Breuer she told about her father's early disease symptoms witch taking her symptoms gradually decreased until she was cured. Breuer started to refer this type of patients to Freud. In the book "Studien uber hysterie" 1895 describes Freud and Breuer a number of interesting cases and begins to use the terms displacement and the unconscious in order to explain the reasons to the hysterical symptoms and also to sexual factors may be behind. Freud believed that in order to be able to treat hysterical patients so was he forced to listen and understand the stories and leave hypnosis as a treatment. Instead he let the patients do free associating lying in sofa with Freud sitting behind and analyzing causes for the illness. This led to the development of psychoanalysis as a working method.

Interesting from this time is that Sweden's Queen Viktoria hired Axel Munthe from 1903 to her death in 1930 as her personal physician, among other things during their stays on the island Capri during the winter season. Axel Munthe who built the famous Villa San Michele in the village of Anacapri has in his book "the book of San Michele" several chapters which deal with the use of hypnosis. Munthe was well acquainted with Charots Tuesday lectures in which hypnosis was before invited audiences and had even visited the Nancy school where Bernheim treated their patients with suggestion methods. In the book describes Munthe that hypnosis was effective where other methods proved to be inactive as treatment of , among other thing alcoholism, morphisms and other dependencies. Munthe that took part as English Red Cross doctor during the first world war in Flanders 1915 gives an account of how he , with the help of hypnosis could provide analgesia for hurt soldiers then morphine and chloroform had ended up . Munthe, who from the beginning was studying Gynecology worked later as the nervous doctor first in Paris during the 1880 's and then in Rome in the 1890 's and describes how hypnosis was used in the treatment of mainly upper-class women in his practice.

The modern hypnosis development

During the twentieth century so has the development of hypnosis continued with, among other things Clark Leonard Hull (1884-1952) who was an experimental psychiatrist, which in later years interested himself for "behavioral psychology" but that in the beginning of his career researching in experimental hypnosis at Yale University and published in 1933 a scientific book "Hypnosis and Suggestibility" which contained detailed studies of the phenomenon of hypnosis with detailed statistical analysis. Hulls report was the first comprehensive scientific study of hypnosis had large influence on the continuation of hypnosis-research.

Finally in this short history description of hypnosis development where many influential scientists not been affected may be mentioned the American Milton Erickson (1901-1980) who is one of the twentieth century's Giants when it comes to work with practical Hypnotherapy. Erickson's major contribution is to give indirect suggestions through regular calls during hypnosis therapy. Erickson was an expert on the intuitive uses all avenues to influence the patient such as their favorite words, cultural background, neurotic habits, and personal history accommodation. Erickson pointed out that the unconscious mind is separated from consciousness and has its own consciousness, interests, reaction patterns and learning. He believed that the unconscious mind was creative, resolve problem and often positive. It has formed a special Erickson tradition where many hypnosis therapist use terms such as confusion and metaphors to reach and affect the patient's unconscious minds.

Today's use of hypnosis involves both clinical use in Psychiatry and analgesia in certain types of surgery or dentistry.

Susceptibility of hypnosis treatment

When it comes to the ability to hypnotize people, show research that about 10% are highly susceptible to hypnosis, while 5-10% is not susceptible to hypnosis. The other 80-85% of the population is in different degree susceptible to hypnosis. In order to determine in the degree to which a person is susceptible to hypnosis, it has established a number of standardized ways to measure the degree of hypnosis deep of a prospective patient or subject. There are two different standards that become common, on the other hand, the Stanford Hypnotic Susceptibility Scale (SHSS) from 1959 for the measurement of individual persons and part Harvard Group Scale (HGSS) from 1962 when the case of groups. Here shows the different steps according to the Stanford Hypnotic Susceptibility Scale (SHSS). The scale was defined by hypnosis researcher Andre Weizenhoffer and Enerst Hilgard in 1959 and has been revised several times referred to as A, B, and C release.

In the SHSS: C is defined the following steps where it gradually puts a person in an ever deepening hypnosis state and check that the correct hypnosis deep is obtained in each state.

0 Eye closure

1 Hand lowering

2 Moving hand apart

3 Mosquito hallucination

4 Taste hallucinations

5 Arm rigidity (right arm)

6 Dreams

7 Age regression (school)

8 Arm immobilization envisaged

9 Anosmia to ammonia

10 Hallucinated voice

11 Negative visual hallucination (three boxes)

12 Post hypnotic amnesia

First step means that the person goes to easy hypnosis and his eyes closing automatically. Step 12, the largest hypnosis depth, means that you can give post hypnotic suggestions during the hypnosis that people perform after waking up without knowing why and to total amnesia about what had happened during the hypnosis. Other conditions are described in the document SHSS: C and procedure takes a total of about 50 minutes.

There have been a number of research studies which examined the differences between the brain activity of people that are easy to put in the hypnotic state and those who are difficult to hypnotize. Professor of Psychiatry David Spiegel at Stanford Center for integrative medicine has led a study where 12 subjects who are easy to hypnotize and 12 persons who are difficult to hypnotize have been investigated with brain scan (fMRI), which investigated which parts of the brain that are affected during the hypnosis state. In the report "Functional Brain Basis of Hypnotizability" published by "Archives of General Psychiatry" (see ref. 8.1) reported the results of the study. The researchers examined brain activity in three different important networks in the brain part "default-mode network" (sleep network) which is active in the rest when no external stimuli affect the brain, on the other hand, "executive control network" which is active in decision making and on the other hand, "the salience network" which is active in prioritize between impressions to select the most important decision making base. Studies of magnetic x-ray camera (fMRI) showed that both groups had a similar active "default-mode network" but the people who had high susceptibility to hypnosis had more corporations between the "executive control network" and "salience network". Especially as these people had an activity in "left dorsolateral prefrontal cortex" in the "executive control" region of the brain in parallel with the "dorsal anterior cingulate cortex in " salience network which plays role in focusing of attention's. The group with low hypnosis sensitivity had little interaction between these networks. Dr. Spiegel notes that the study confirms that hypnosis sensitivity is of small extent depends on the person's personal characteristics but more dependent on cognitive sensitivity. Dr. Spiegel also points out that the study shows a clear difference in brain activity between people who easily can be hypnotized, and those that are difficult to hypnotize.

Hypnosis state may affect the experience of all senses as hearing, sight, touch, smell and taste, but the extent depends on the person's ability to achieve different hypnosis depth. The English psychiatrist John Hartland gives in his book "Clinical hypnosis", 1974; examples of different ways to affect the experience of sensory input during the Hypnosis (see ref. 8.2).

When it comes to our vision can a hypnotic suggestion get the person to become partially or totally blind. Also the influence of color can be done so that the subject looks in a black and white image or affect color experience. At measurement of EEG waves for a person who suggested not being able to see, can be seen brainwaves that is the same as those from a blind person or a person with closed eyes. When it comes to hearing can, as already found by the James Braid at hypnosis experiment, hearing is tightened much under hypnosis. It is believed that intervention is partly due to the fact that the hypnotized have disabled all external sensory stimulation, relevant and focused solely on your hearing. Like as for the vision, you can give the hypnotized to become totally deaf. You can unexpectedly fire a rifle behind the person whiteout that he hears something or react with elevated blood pressure. When you suggest a hypnotized person of deafness, it is necessary to instruct the person to the hypnosis is interrupted by a character or for example touch of the shoulder or to not interrupt the hypnosis with a spoken command. The deafness or blindness that was suggested in hypnosis state is a psychological phenomenon. Senses perform their usual functions but impressions and irritations can't reach up to consciousness.

When it comes to the smell so can you also by suggestion during hypnosis sharpening the sense of smell, but also reduce or turn off the sense of smell so as not to feel the stinging fumes from, for example ammonia, which is one of the tests of hypnosis depth 9 of the previously described SHSS scale. Similarly, it is possible to strengthen or weaken the taste during hypnosis. You can get the complete absence of flavor so that a strong chili fruit becomes tasteless or for example any suggestion to plain water gets a sweet or bitter taste. Even touching can by suggestion during hypnosis affected so that the sensitivity to pain is reduced or wiped out entirely (analgesia).

For the approximately 10 % of the population that can be put in the deep hypnotic trance or somnambular trance, can hallucinations be developed that is totally alien and inexplicable. People who reach somnambular trance, for example open his eyes and still be in trance and continues to carry out the suggestions that hypnotist give. During this deep trance, you can give people to see hallucinations, perform complex posthypnotic suggestions, become insensitive to pain and having complete amnesia (loss of memory) for what has happened during the trance after waking up. When it comes to illusions (incorrect perception of an objective fact) or hallucinations (perception of an object or person, where no is present) so can these people be given suggestions to for which any of the five senses perceive positive or negative illusions or hallucinations. Positive hallucinations mean that the hypnotized person suggested seeing a person or objecting that does not exist. The negative hallucinations means suggestion that you cannot see a particular person or object, which can be heard in that if the hypnotist hands a cigarette packet to the third person, as the hypnotized not can see, so think he that cigarette package available in thin air.

In addition to the five senses hypnosis has the ability to affect the body's other features like muscle, the autonomic nervous system and other biochemical changes in the body. When it comes to volitional controlled muscles so can hypnosis affect muscles to become quite lax and can bring paralysis in i.e. an arm muscle. It is possible to put the body's muscles in catalepsy which can make the body completely stiff so that the person can be laid with the support of only two chairs at the shoulder and one at the feet. In addition, provide increased muscle strength and influence the automatic movements. The autonomic nervous system can with hypnosis affecting for example blood circulation, breathing, digestion and endocrine glands for the treatment of psychosomatic diseases. Through hypnosis, the tiny capillary blood vessels made to retract, which can reduce blood flow in operations, damage or dentist treatment. Hypnosis can also cause reactions in the skin, so that for example a hypnosis experiment in which an ordinary pen is pressed against the skin and a suggestion is given if that it is hot may afterwards develop burn blow even though no heat were added. Hypnosis has also been used for to alleviate allergic skin reactions and restore the smooth skin.

Hypnosis and pain relief

As was mentioned in the historical development of hypnosis it is a compelling phenomenon that during deep hypnotic trance so can analgesia (pain relief) even be total under surgery interventions without any form of chemical anesthesia. This can lead to leg amputated, breast operation and dental operations can be carried out without any toxic side effects from the anesthetic. Even under a hypnotic deep trance, you can use hypnosis to reduce the use of anesthetic and often shortened in addition, rehabilitation time and aftercare. There are many studies in the field of surgical care where you found hypnosis improved effect on the patient's experience and recovery.

Examples of surgical care with hypnosis is provided in a study "Breast cancer surgery under hypnosis and local anesthesia: Feasibility and potential benefits" from professor Fabienne Roelants and Dr. Christine Watremez from Belgium. The study refers to the use of hypnosis for breast cancer surgery and thyroid surgery (see ref. 8.3). In breast cancer study attended 78 patients, of whom 18 patients were treated with hypnosis and local anesthesia while the rest received treatment with regular anesthesia methods. While hypnosis patients needed a longer time in the operating room, so reducing the need for opioid anesthesia and they had less time for aftercare and total hospitalization time. In thyroid operations group included 36 patients with common anesthesia methods and 18 patients who got a local anesthetic and hypnosis treatment. The result of these operations showed again that the hypnosis treatment reduced patients ' need for anesthetics and the need for aftercare and total hospitalization decreased radically. Professor Roelants stressed that in breast cancer surgery under hypnosis, so gives also anesthetic drug to reduce stress during operation and may reduce the risk of cancer spread. The result of the study is that about 33 % of thyroid operations and 25 % of breast cancer operations at UCL hospital, so used local anesthetic in Combination with hypnosis treatment. The method improves the patient's experience of the operation and reduces the total cost of hospitalization.

Even in Sweden, among other things at the Swedish Medical University Karolinska Institutet have operations with only hypnosis carried out. In the newspaper Aftonbladet 2009-04-30 sets out for a patient, that is typically feel bad of anesthesia and general anesthesia, in which a pacemaker was replaced in hypnosis treatment. During the operation was hypnotist Camilla Jansson-Rönning with and gave induction during the hypnosis. The patient felt no pain and nurses mentioned that heart sounds and blood pressure was unusually stable during operation.

Hypnosis state can also affect the person's memory functions. In the context of the trials used hypnosis to try to access the forgotten memories of the often traumatic blasphemy at the crime. Sometimes, repressed details captured in hypnosis session, but it is very restrictive when using this result as evidence at court. Experiments with people who are easy to get in deep hypnosis has also shown that you can plant into false memories during the hypnosis with suggestions that the person cannot distinguish from true perceived events after waking up from hypnosis state.

You often hear associated with hypnosis demonstrations to hypnotist indicates that it is not against their will can be made to do things that the hypnotist give. According to a number of sources such as: in the researcher Barbara Brown's book "The hidden power" (see ref. 7.1) writes she " The most highly educated hypnotizers and many scene hypnotizers as well, claiming that the commandments to Act on a certain way does not work if the individual's opinions are in contradiction to the action. The common example is that you are not able to get a person during hypnosis to commit one crime therefore to personal and cultural morality is too deep fixed in the individual's subconscious mind. Baloneys how can a hypnotized person who holds on to carry out their orders to make a distinction between an opinion and a different? A human being can be asked to kill another human being for their country's sake when it's war because of his/her views is such, but if a hypnotized succeeded and the subject trust on hypnotist enough lot for to put himself and breastfeed a per shoes or close of the pain when surgery inserts in them (which indeed is contrary to one's social performance), then is it obvious that during hypnosis very dramatically can change people's opinions or faiths. "

I read already in 1960's the book "Hypnosis", by the psychologist and the neurologist F. L. Marcuse (see ref. 8.4) which appeared as professor at the State College of Washington, which in a whole chapter 8 "will issue and the moral question "analyzes the ability to get people to do things against their will under deep hypnosis and notes that it doesn't is so easy to answer. Marcuse says in a summary conclusion "That have been reported too many positive result for that we would dare to suggest that antisocial actions impossible can be made during hypnosis. For its own part would I certainly did not want to serve as a test subject in an experiment that completely optimistic took answer no for granted. The question whether the experimenter or the object should be made responsible for an immoral action be cartoon I as a legal problem rather than as a psychological, and I said me assumed that the as conducts the action (the hypnotized) rather than hypnotist would be found wanting to blame if it was tried before a judge. ---The Question about whether or not someone under hypnosis can be induced to do something which goes against his (or her) moral principles are inappropriately worded and must be written about, so that it in rather than get the following wording: Can someone under hypnosis induced to do something that is social and objectively culpable? If the question is formulated in this way, is the answer according to my opinion- Yes."

In TV channel Discovery Science has it aired a program about hypnosis in the series "Curiosity: Brainwashed" under the title "What is hypnosis" where one out of a group of 185 people gradually picked out people who could go into the depth of hypnosis and finally elected a person out of the final experiment. In the program involved several scientists among others memory researcher Cynthia Meyersburg at Harvard university, Tom Silver which is a certified hypnotherapist and psychologist Jeff Kieiszenski that comments on and monitor the experiment. Volunteers are given suggestions under deep hypnosis on to a designated person is a dangerous terrorist who have wound up at a designated post hypnotic command. A faked situation outside a hotel arranged and volunteers receive a bag with a gun with blanks and given the post hypnotic command. The program ends with the subject shoot target person with the fake weapon. The program was also to the assassination of Robert Kennedy in June 1968, where the attempt man Sirhan B Sirhan shot the Kennedy. Sirhan was sentenced to life imprisonment but defense lawyers have tried to prove that Sirhan was hypnotized during the attack and that a conspiracy was behind the assassination.

A different use of hypnosis is to bring a person gradually back in time through suggest regression. In cases where real regression to i.e. 5 year age, so move the person to a previous stage of development and has forgotten everything that happen later in life. Ask the person to write his name, so similar to the type style in the person's old school books. Even the person's speech and behavior is on a 5-year-old's level, where he can tell profanity from this period. Through hypnotic regression can be very unconscious mental and emotional conflicts that are behind neurological disease. In other cases, successful person not really return to the previous stage of development but the browser itself as he believes that a child in the age group behaves. But even in this case, the memories come up that the person does not remember in his usual adult liv.

Theories on hypnosis state

It is still difficult to fully explain how a hypnotic trance and the mechanisms that affects the brain's different centers of perception and interpretation of how the brain's networks are involved. Hypnosis is dependent of the person's sensitivity to how suggestions are processed in the brain.

Generally it can be said that the unconscious mind is strongly including under hypnosis induction. You could say the following about the unconscious impact during hypnotic trance:

• Suggestion affects the person much stronger if it appears in the unconscious mental life.

• Critical ability is under hypnosis is wholly or partly inhibited.

• Under certain circumstances the unconscious fill almost all the conciseness features, with the exception of the critical ability (compare system 1 in Chapter 5 about intuition).

• When suggestions bypass the conscious, which is under the hypnosis penetrates directly into the unconscious, which has little or no capacity for criticism and therefore cannot reject it, why the person must act according to it.

In hypnosis research, there are different theories about how the hypnotic trance occurs and if hypnosis state is a State of consciousness separate from the normal consciousness. There are two schools in hypnosis research that either says that hypnosis is a trance state or an altered state of consciousness in the brain (State theories), while others believe that there is a social psychological reason to hypnosis (Non-state theories) and believe that hypnosis is not something unique permission but can occur without hypnotic induction or trance. In coarse features, the differences in the approach are described in table 8.1.

Table 8.1 Different theories of hypnosis

State teories	Non-State teories
Hypnotic induction gives an altered state of consciousness in the brain.	Participants react to suggestions as well without hypnosis.
Hypnotic trance is associated with an altered function in the brain.	Participants in hypnosis experiment are actively engaged.
The response of hypnotic suggestions is the result of special processes in the brain that dissociation or altered state of consciousness.	Response to suggestion is a product of normal psychology processes that attitude, expectations and motivation.
Hypnotic susceptibility is an-labelling worth stable over long period.	Suggestions sensitivity can be altered by drugs and psychological impact.

None of the proposed theories can alone explain the hypnosis state and it's probably unrealistic to a single psychological mechanism can provide the entire declaration. You can see several components that are involved in the hypnotic phenomena such as: quality of the hypnotic induction (affects memory, relaxation and alertness), depth of hypnotic state (hypnotic susceptibility, dissociation and susceptibility) and the hypnotic suggestion natural (intensity and clarity).

With modern methods such as EEG and magnetic imaging (fMRI), is it possible in hypnosis research today to measure the different parts of the brain that are affected during the hypnosis experiment. A research team at University of Skövde, Sweden, in the direction of Sakari Kallio in cooperation with Turku University in Finland has conducted two studies, on the other hand, a study of eye movements during hypnotic trance 2011 and, on the other hand, a study of altered color experience during hypnotic trance in 2013.

The study of eye movements is published in Kallio S, Hyönä J, Revonsuo A, Sikka P, Nummenmaa L, 2011, "The Existence of Hypnotic State Revealed by Eye Movements" (see ref. 8.5). The trial was carried out so that the subject had to see three different kinds of images on a 21 " monitor. The first task was to fix the gaze at a point in the middle of the picture for 5 seconds and the background was varied in four steps from black to 90 % white randomly. The researchers used an advanced "eye tracker" which measured several parameters such as number of eye fixations, number of blinks, pupil lens size and eyes fixation time for that document the eye movements during hypnosis trials. The subject was a 43 year old woman who is very receptive to hypnosis with the value 12 at SHSS: C scale for hypnosis depth which is characterized by the ability to total amnesia and hallucinations during hypnosis. During the trials, the subject turned to hypnosis directly caused a glassy stare look but also a strong change in auto reflective range of eye movements. The result was compared at measurements with a control group of 14 persons, who were instructed to try to fake the corresponding eye movements' as imitate the hypnotic effect on the subject. The report showed that hypnotically induced glassy gaze of the subject was followed by large, objective and non-imitate changes in the subject's eye movements in which amplitude, speed and frequency was radically less while fixation time increased. Even pupil size decreased during hypnosis. The conclusion of the study is that it is a first demonstration of the existence of a special hypnotic state resulting from the empirical criteria for such a permit (immediate induction and immobilize, objective confirmation by measuring and non-imitate in normal condition).

Study on altered color experience under hypnosis is published in Koivisto M, Kirjanen S, Revonsuo A, Kallio 's, 2013 "A Preconscious Neural Mechanism of Hypnotically Altered Colors: A Single Case Study" (see ref.8.6). The trial were carried out through that on a monitor present three geometrical forms tringle, circle and square random in red or blue color with one figure in a time for the trial subjects. Their task was to identify characters ' color. Over attempts were documented brain activities with EEG equipment. Two subjects which were very susceptible to hypnosis, on the other hand, the same woman who took part in earlier described eye movement study with the value 12 at SHSS: C scale and a 40 year old woman with the value 9 at SHSS: C scale. During hypnosis trail so was the subjects served a post hypnotic suggestion to one of the characters, for example that all squares are red, before the experiment started. The first subject was completely influenced by the suggestion and reported squares as red even when they were blue. The researchers discovered that when a figure that included in the monitor appeared suggestion, so you could see a high level of high-frequency activity in the EEG curves after a 1/10 second in her brain. The other woman volunteers could not experience the color changing but reported a strange phenomenon in connection with the mentioned suggestion "sometimes, I felt a strange feeling that my eyes said that some characters have a certain color but my brain told me that there was another color". The high-frequency activity in the brain of the first volunteers is considered to reflect a situation when the brain automatically compares the incoming information with in-formation that already exists in memory. In this case, could it in hypnosis give a very strong memory (that all squares are red) which then automatically became activated when a square appeared on the screen. Of this subject was suggestion so strong that it could replace the square right color. The results show that the first test subject hallucinating colors fully automatically and unconsciously during hypnosis. When the subject did try that with the help of imagination cause the same changes without hypnosis so could she not. Sari Kallio notes that this study shows that hypnotic behavior can be completely automatic and caused by processes in the brain that you are unaware of.

Today used hypnosis as a tool for clinical treatments in many different areas such as phobias (i.e. fear of flying, snake horror), post-traumatic stress condition, smoking cessation, weight reduction, etc. and is a recognized medical treatment. In 1955, it approved "The British Medical Association" (BMA) official use of hypnosis for psychics' neuroses and for pain relief during surgery and birth. In the United States in 1958 approved "The American Medical Association (AMA) use of hypnosis, after which "The American Psychological Association" recognized hypnosis as a branch of psychology.

This chapter shows that hypnosis, which is part of the book's concept "The Unconscious Zone", can influence the unconscious in the brain functions in a powerful way. 90 % of the population can be affected by hypnosis in varying degrees, of which about 10% can reach the deepest hypnosis trance, where the full pain relief (analgesia) during even that an operation can be done. Clinical activities with hypnosis can be effective on many areas such as the treatment of phobia, smoking cessation, weight reduction, etc. Much research about the behind mechanisms in the brain goes on, among other things in Sweden, where the new methods with EEG and magnetic imaging (fMRI) brings with it the opportunity to measure the brain network involved in hypnosis state. Recent research at the University of Skövde, Sweden points to the possibility of a deep hypnosis state causes an altered State of consciousness in the brain that underpins State theories of hypnosis trance.

Chapter 9 Placebo, nocebo

The power of thoughts

Placebo effect is a reality in connection with any provision of medical treatment, but then it is a strong positive expectation force so it can be said that it is active also in e.g. professional life where a strong faith on a project or professional role can be decisive for success. The opposite is called nocebo and have a negative impact on medical treatment and could even be in voodoo magic context develop fatal influence of a vulnerable person. The designations placebo and nocebo is used in the literature mainly regarding the medical treatment of diseases, but in the continued production will also other forms of mental psychological influence of the human body can be affected. It should be noted that, today in a holistic thinking, cannot distinguish psyche from the body but we must see the symbiotic relationship mind/body which directly depending of each other. The heading of the chapter, the power of thoughts, refers to communicating with the mind versus Body (Body/Mind), placebo effects strongly attached to the patient's thoughts and desires. This underlines the phrase that "faith can put a mountain". Research also shows that placebo effects can also influence a patient on an unconscious level in "The Unconscious Zone".

Placebo, nocebo effects

In the TV program "Placebo" in science's world (SVT October 2013), were shown two telling examples of the two different effects of placebo and nocebo. The first example of a placebo is a case that occurs during the Second World War during the fighting in the spring of 1944 at mountain Monte Cassino in Italy, where the Allied forces were attacked during the intensive bombardment of a German attack. The attack resulted in many damaged Allied soldier, who were put on stretchers in long rows in the tent that served as a field hospital. Many had severe pain from the sores lesions in different body parts. When the anesthesia doctor Henry Beecher just would start to operate an injured soldier so discovered that it was a lack of morphine in the medicine supply. In desperation took he and the Assistant nurse the drastic decision to give the wounded soldier an injection with normal saline, but pretended that it was a syringe with morphine. The nurse assured the patient that he would soon feel the pain is alleviated. The soldier's expectation to get morphine had enabled his brains receptors in the opioid system and signals went through the spine and stopped pain signals so that they are not reaching the brain. Then he already previously received morphine for pain relief had the soldier the same expectations as this time enabled the opioid system and sent out endorphin which is an endogenous effective pain relief.

This incident appeared to further research on placebo effect started in the 1940s by the anesthesia doctor Henry Beecher, which was physician in the US Army and served as Lieutenant Colonel both in North Africa and in the related attack in Italy. Dr. Beecher that from the beginning, surgery worked from 1939 as Chief of anesthesia training at Harvard Medical School and became professor in the specialty in 1941, before he was called up for service in the army during the Second World War. Beecher returned to Harvard Medical School after the war and focused them on to examine the experiences of placebo effect into which he saw with the wounded soldiers on war battlefields and published the book "Pain in Man Wounded in the Battle". In the book he outlined for the experience of war that severely injured soldiers did not feel pain despite that they not received treatment until after several hours.

Beecher started the research with clinical studies to document the placebo effects. Beecher published an article in "The Journal of the American Medical Association in 1955 under the title " The Powerful Placebo "(Ref. 9.1) and described how placebo effect rejects the results of dozens of experiments with new drugs. He gave an account of the subjects who received medicine also got placebo effects of to take the pills which therapeutic increased the medical effect. He stated that it is only by subtracting effects of placebo you can see how drug's own positive effect operate.

The article got a big impact within the medical profession, but in spite of Beecher's purposeful work to introduce better experimental models in pharmaceutical tests took it to 1962 before the Congress introduced a law Food, Drug and Cosmetic ACT (FDA). The reason for the law was among other things that man received injuries in newborn children depends on the drug side effects and wanted to achieve better security against side effects and that called for control groups with placebo treatment to document that the drug had desired effect. Before the law was introduced was performed many pharmaceutical tests through to increase the dose until the subjects had side effects of the medicine and then was elected a lower therapeutic concentration. Beecher's contribution was to suggest that pharmaceutical tests would be carried out partly double-blind (neither doctors nor patient knows who that received the placebo), a comparison group of patients treated with placebo (sugar pill) and selection to placebo or active funds would occur randomly. The FDA ruled also that in order for a drug to be approved to get better results than a placebo pill and that at least two independent studies have been carried out. The law got a radical influence on pharmaceutical companies and showed that a part previously approved drugs probably not had been approved with the new requirements.

Second example involving nocebo effect was raised by Giuliana Mazzoni who is professor of psychology at the University of Hull as report about a case in which a young man who suffered from depression, took part in a clinical trial of an antidepressant drug, a double blind test, in which neither the researchers nor the patient knew what that got the drug or placebo (sugar pill). The patient felt that the antidepressant pills worked well and he became less depressed. Then happen it a case that the relationship with his girlfriend took out and he fell back in in a deeper depression. He then took the drastic decision to commit suicide and decided to pass on to empty all the medicine bottle of tablets which he receives from the clinical trial. He felt that the overdose lowered his blood pressure to a dangerous level and the internal organ began to shut down. He was taken in an ambulance to an emergency room, where they saw very serious on the patient's condition. The blood tests showed that one could not see any poisoning of the drugs, why the doctor wanted to get to the bottom of the case then something obviously was wrong. After contact with the responsible researcher for the clinical trial there was showed that the patient had been given placebo pills and then overdosed on sugar pills and held nevertheless on to die. His life was saved but how could he get in this state of sugar pills? The case shows how a nocebo effect has arisen out of the patient's expectations by taking an overdose of highly effective medicine (he has in the past been less depressed by medicine) and thus set in motion powerful movements in his body which had an impact on the autonomic nervous system. They say that belief can puts mountains and research shows that faith and expectations is one of the foundations of placebo/nocebo effects.

Modern placebo research

One of the researchers that during the 1990's interest in itself for the mechanism behind the placebo/nocebo effect are Fabrizio Benedetti who is a professor of Physiology and Neurology at the University of Turine at the Faculty of medicine, Italy. Many believe that Benedetti is behind that research on placebo has received increasing interest even in the pharmaceutical industry and that his institution is a world leader in the research branch. Benedetti published 2008 a book "Placebo Effects: Understanding the mechanisms in health and disease" (see ref. 9.2), which garnered a great deal of interest in the new research in the placebo/nocebo area.

In an article "The many placebo effects" (Ref. 9.3), 2011, describes Benedetti for a number of mechanisms that underlie the placebo effects as expectations, learning and genetic influences. Placebo effect is basically a psycho biological process in which treatment with inactive pills (sugar pills), inactive injections (saline), acupuncture with non-penetrating needles and fictitious operations including verbal psychological stimulation found to have effect on a patient's experience of treatment and in many cases provides up to 50% reduction of pain sensation. At nocebo effects can negative influence of information about potential side effects of inert pills or treatments affect the patient to be aware of these disorders even though the pills are completely inactive (sugar pill). These effects must be addressed in the context of medical tests of new drugs when the results might otherwise be misleading.

Research in the placebo/nocebo effect of pain management sets great demands on to isolate response from placebo mechanisms from the often natural variations in ongoing medical conditions. In figure 9.1 shows a basic picture of the different mechanisms that can affect the patient's experience of pain associated with various medical conditions. Here some differences that can affect the results from a treatment.

• An impact may be due to a particular disease can spontaneous healing or fluctuating symptoms in relapse, which can occur while a placebo treatment begins. A way to exclude this mechanism is to have a reference group which is not dealt with actively in order to be able to compare the results of this effect.

• Regression to the mean is a statistical phenomenon dependent on the inaccuracies in the selection.

• The patient or the physician's classification of pain experience may include inaccuracies in the estimation of a pain level. Even differences in patients ' experiences of pain level can play into drug tests.

• Any errors in the physician's diagnosis of the disease.

• Side effects, such as when a placebo injection is provided so can effect of lurch from when the needle penetrates the skin indirectly result in a reduction of the pain experience.

Below are reported the placebo/nocebo effects into which you want to be within explore and map out psychosocial and psychobiological impact.

• The influence of genetic factors on the placebo response.

• Influence through expectancy in brain systems that manage the patient's anxiety in the face of medical treatment on the placebo response.

• Influence over the expectation in the brain's reward systems (dopamine system) of the placebo response.

• Influence through condition reflexes according to Pavlov on placebo response.

• Influence through social contacts, where e.g. others ' experiences of treatment affect.

• Influence over the previous own treatments confirming the treatment result.

Fig. 9.1 Placebo effects

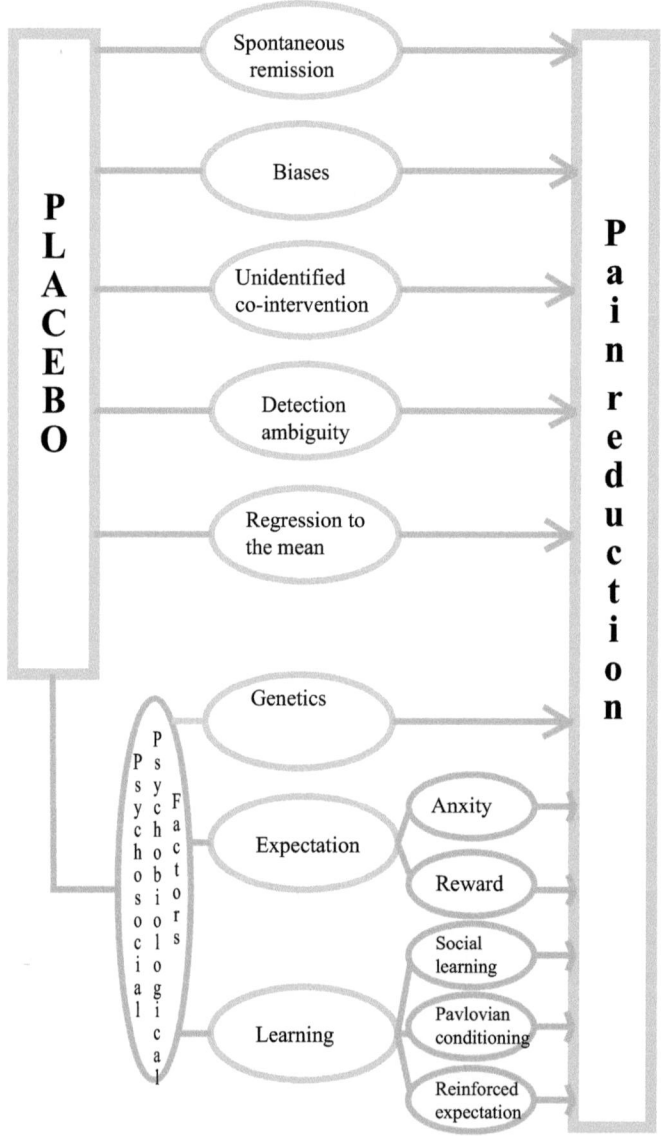

According to Benedetti is the best way to document the placebo/ nocebo effects find synergies to study pain state or Parkinson›s disease, because the neural networks that affect these conditions in large part has been identified. The mechanism involves opioid-CCK-dopamine networks that affect pain and parts of the basal ganglia network in question about Parkinson›s disease. Important conclusions have been drawn about the placebo/nocebo effects in studies of these neural networks.

In usual clinical tests are only interested to establish whether it tried the drug has a better influence on the illness than the inactive agent in placebo pills. But in the case of review of real antidepressant pharmaceutical tests (Kirsch in «listening to Prozac but hearing placebo: a metaanalysis of antidepressant medication») (see ref. 9.4) has been able to show that 25 % of patients have rated a spontaneous healing and to 50% have received a mere placebo effect while only 25% of patients have a real influence of the drug. In his book «The emperor›s new drugs: Exploring the antidepressant myth» (see ref. 9.5) describes the psychology professor Irwing Kirsch how the pharmaceutical industry in its eagerness to get new drugs approved by FDA, using methods for to get medicines to appear in a better light by not publishing negative study, publish the same positive studies several times, publish selectively from some study, publish data that distinguishes itself from the reports to the FDA and made repeated test until you got a positive result.

General information about the mechanisms of placebo effect is the patient›s expectations on the treatment of disease that must be initiated. Generally, said that expectations are a way for the body to predict and manage an expected result of the treatment. A mechanism is to expect negative results of medical treatment increases the concern and thus pain, while an expected positive results reduces the pain and enable the reward system in the body. In studies it has been shown that during placebo treatment so have the patient›s anxiety is reduced depending on that when the patient expects that the pain should subside shortly, reduces anxiety and thus reduces the activation of brain areas that deal with concern and threat for example the amygdala, which are involved in pain perceptions.

Survey of the patient›s anxiety depends on a person›s personal orientation or worry/anxiety in a particularly vulnerable situation shows that placebo affect at pain perception is reduced during an acute stress condition, while if the patient have a nervous personality is not placebo effective. Even in Sweden are carried out research on the placebo/nocebo effect at the Karolinska Institutet (KI) in Stockholm under the direction of Martin Ingvar who is a professor of the Department of integrative medicine. The research is funded by a donation in 2005 from an American businessman Bernard Osher called «the Osher Centre for Integrative Medicine». The Institute conducts research projects in various complementary medical treatments such as acupuncture, sleep problem, hypnosis and the placebo/ nocebo effects.

There are a number of research papers from Institute on placebo effects, where, among other things researcher Dr. Predrag Petrovic studied placebo effects with PET and fMRI methods. At study with the help of fMRI of brain activities worry/anxiety network (see Predrag Petrovic, et al, «Placebo in emotional processing induced expectations of anxiety relief activate a generalized modulatory network", Ref. 9.6) can you see a declining effect of discomfort depending on the placebo effects.

At this experiment the first day got healthy subjects the drug Midazolam (benzodiazepine) or benzodiazepine receptor antagonist Flumazenil in connection with presentation of images with strong shocking/objectionable content (e.g. mutilated bodies). As expected relaxed Midazolam effect at the presentation of the unpleasant images while Flumazenil had opposed increasing effect of discomfort. After the first day had subject›s expectations has been strengthened to respond on the two different medicines. When the experiment went on day two people were informed that they would receive the same treatment by drugs, but instead got the placebo treatment with verbal information about the medicinal product contained the same substance that during day one. It was a significant result which placebo gave the same results as Midazolam with reduction of unease the sense when you entered that the drug was given, while it was increased discomfort when the antagonist Flumazenil was specified as medicines in placebo. Study with

216

fMRI showed that blood flow in the brain was changed both in the anterior cingulate cortex (ACC) and lateral orbitofrontal cortex (see fig. 9.2), witch areas also are involved in placebo analgesia. In a previous study (Petrovic P, Kalso E, Pettersson KM, Ingvar M, 2002, «Placebo and opioid analgesia imaging a shard neuronal network, Ref. 9.7») with PET methods were shown to the same neural net-work involved in pain management using morphine also is involved in placebo treatment with a placebo injection of saline solution in which the body›s own pain relieving endorphins is involved. Studies point to that it is similar to mechanisms that are included in the placebo effect at the emotional impact as the analgesic effects via the placebo pills/injections (expectation). In addition to expectations and learning to have some research indicated that some genetic components can influence the placebo effects as in for example psychiatric diseases, depression and panic attacks.

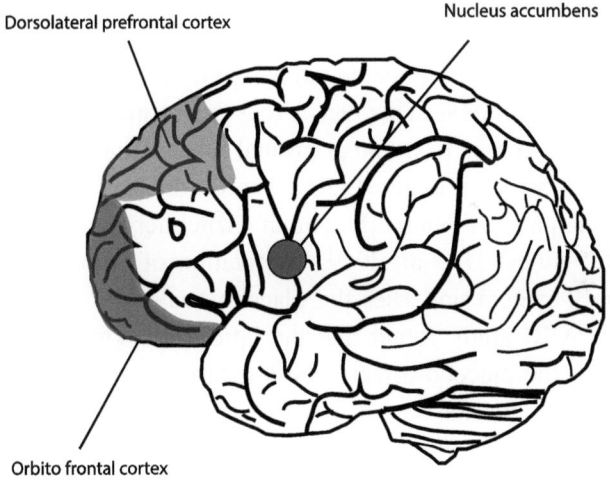

Fig. 9.2 Anatomy placebo areas

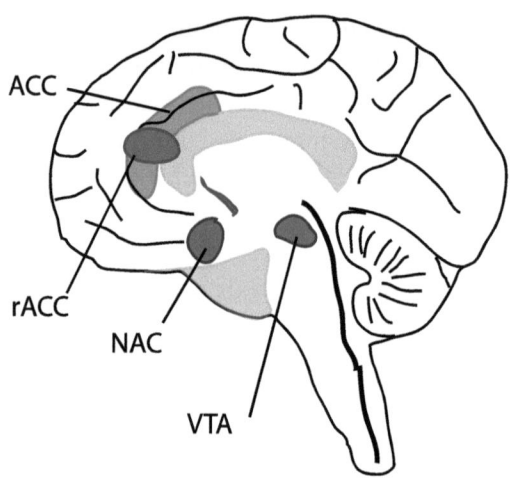

Fig. 9.3 Anatomy Nucleus accumbens

Benedetti has even in studies with the help of, among other things EEG analysis found that patients with Alzheimer's disease have a reduced ability to get any placebo response. EEG analyses showing that an Alzheimer's patient has a degenerated neural network between the prefrontal lobes and to other brain areas. This means that the normal expectation effect of placebo which comes from the prefrontal lobes do not reach out to opioid network, why we have to give higher doses of such as morphine in order to get the same pain relieving effect of an Alzheimer's patient. Other studies (Eippert F, Bingel U et al, 2009, "Activation of opioidergic descending pain control system underlies the placebo analgesia", Ref. 9.8 ") where man with fMRI study found that the opioid blocking antagonist naloxone reduces the placebo effect dorsolateral prefrontal induced from cortex and rostral anterior cingulate cortex (rACC). These two mechanisms with blockade of placebo induced pain relief from Alzheimer's disease and from opioid antagonist naloxone from prefrontal lobes can also in the experiment are developed with repetitive Transcranial Magnetic Stimulation (rTMS) of prefrontal cortex. This point strongly to the prefrontal lobes of the brain is involved in placebo effects.

218

When it comes to nocebo effect, there is also research that shows that worry/anxiety network is involved in increasing pain impact. In one study (Colla L, Sisaudo M, Benedetti F, 2008, The role of learning in nocebo and placebo effects, ref. 9.9) with healthy people who were given either a tactile or electrical pain generated by a low-intensity shock pain could be strengthened through to give an placebo pills with a verbal information to the drug could give an increasing pain perception. It was therefore a nocebo effect which can give increasing pain perception and also for example some areas of skin can be painful highly responsive to touch. Negative expectations of a treatment can give a reinforcement of pain conditions in several of brain regions that deal with pain, as the cingulate cortex, prefrontal cortex, Insula and the hippocampus which features nocebo effects.

Already in 1997 conducted Benedetti a study for to identify the biochemical pathways involved in the placebo/nocebo effects (Benedetti F, Amanzio M, Casadio C, Oilaro A, Maggi G, 1997, "Blockade of nocebo hyperalgesia by the cholecystokinin antagonist proglumide", Ref. 9.10) and discovered that it is a neural mechanism that is directly involved in the Nocebo effects. The study was conducted with post-operative patients who had a mild pain and which received an injection that according to the doctor would intensify the pain within 30 minutes. Either got the patient an inactive injection of saline or substance proglumide which block a hormone cholecystokinin (CCK), which in the case of worrying/anxiety causes greater pain sensitivity. When the patient got a saline injection (placebo) increased pain while at proglumide injections so got to no greater pain reaction. Thus when the receptors for the hormone cholecystokinin was blocked so stopped nocebo effect overall.

At a later study 2006 (Benedetti F, Amanzio M, Vighetti S, Asteggiano G, 2006 "The biochemical and neuroendocrine bases of the hyperalgesia nocebo effect", ref. 9. 11) concluded Benedetti that nocebo effects is strongly related to anxiety/worry network. Proglumide is blocking pain receptors by neutralization of the hormone cholecystokinin (CCK), which is responsible for the increased pain sensitivity. But proglumide affected not the secretion of hormone ACTH which gives hyperactivity of the hypothalamic-pituitary-adrenal network at the nocebo effect. Treatment with the drug Diazepam (benzodiazepine) influencing anxiety/worry network directly through both blocking of CCK and reduce of the hormone (ACTH) has a calming effect.

As mentioned earlier, even the brain's reward system, driven by two basic neurotransmitter part dopamine which, among other things impact increased the well-being and on the other hand, serotonin, which has an inhibitory function, involved in placebo effects. An area in the brain nucleus accumbens (NAC) as out-make a part of the basal ganglia (see fig. 9.3) and counts to the limbic system in the brain's reward system and may control from, among other things ventral tegmental area (VTA) and frontal lobe Gyri. Animal studies have shown that NAC produce more dopamine and serotonin reduces under the influence of drugs. It is VTA that produces dopamine and via axons affect NAC but is also involved in opioid network and are affected by heroin and morphine. NAC is involved in mechanisms of drug dependence and even how our emotional state control facial expressions and body language. Research studies of, among other things. ("David J Scott et al," Individual Differences in Reward Responding Explain Placebo-Induced Expectations and effects ", ref. 9.12) indicate that a large placebo effect is associated with increased dopamine and opioid activity of NAC. While a nocebo effect is the opposite with a decrease of dopamine and opioid activity of NAC. The study also points out that the impact of the placebo/nocebo effect via the NAC is affected by different individuals ' sensitivity and physiology which leads to pain relief using placebo varies a lot between different persons. This is a parameter that should be included in the harvesting of human subjects in research projects.

In addition to placebo effects induced by expectations and learning later research showed that one can get placebo effects even of influence on one of the minds unconscious level. In a study: (Karin B Jensen, Martin Ingvar, Jian Kong, et.al. "Nonconscious activation of placebo and nocebo pain response" Ref. 9.13) is one of the experiments found the placebo/nocebo effects that do not depend on cognitive consciousness. Neuroimaging studies showing that brain structures as the striatum and amygdala processes incoming stimuli's before they reach a conscious level and results in non-conscious effect on cognition and behavior.

Placebo by conditioning

Research on placebo effect depends on conditioning according to Pavlov's model is in progress, among other things under the direction of psychology professor Manfred Schedlowski at the University in Essen Germany. Pavlov showed that it could affect the dogs' salivation regarding expected food through to ring the Bell at the same time as the food was served during a period of time. After that could the saliva secrete be developed by simply calling the Bell when the dog's brain programmed to expect food, so called conditioned reflex. Professor Schedlowski has during long time researching in the field of Immunology, among other things regarding how to prevent rejection of transplanted organ, for example hearts, when the donor is not is close related with the who is transplanted. They have previously studied how to influence the body's immune defense in studies on rats.

A medication that was used to reduce the immune system's repellent of new organ is the drug cyclosporine A, which has a sharp immune reduced effect. In experiments with rats, it has been given a sweet drink while they injected the drug into three training periods with breaks in between. Then get the rat a sweet drink but that medicine is not given, but checks of immunological parameters in the blood indicates that you still get a similar influence of immune system only with placebo the sweet drink. The research results show in case of transplantation can drug be reduced with the help of conditioning according to similar principles and thus give rise to fewer side effects. Other research groups have had similar results with other drugs and in cases where you would like to increase the activity of the immune system. Conditioning is a form of associative learning in which to teach the brain in this case attaches a sweet drink to suppression of the immune system. Other experiments with rats have shown that by transplantation of hearts so push organ away within 8-10 days if we do not give any drugs that suppress repellent. The survival of the rat increased to 15 days if the animal had been conditioned in advance with the sweet drink. If you only added 10% of the normal dose medicine to the rats in connection with conditioning than survived 33 % of the rats the experiment. In order to test if you can get the same results on people it has under the leadership of professor Schedlowski a study conducted on human subjects (Schedlowski M et al, 2002, "Behavioral conditioning of immune suppression is possible in humans" Ref. 9.14) and received significant similar results. The study included 34 healthy men who were tested over a two-week period and divided in two groups in which 18 people got the capsules with the drug cyclosporine A, while the other 16 in the control group got pills looked as the same capsules that contained a placebo. The subjects were informed that they would receive the drug during one of the two weeks but not exactly when. All the subjects were given the same treatment with the intake of pharmaceutical capsules two times (12 h) every day for three days at the intake of a beverage with a special eye catching ill green color and with a new flavor of milk flavored with strawberry taste and drops of lavender oil. The strong color and unique taste have a newsworthy for the nervous system for to develop strong cognitive reactions for quick learning. During day 4-7 were given no further treatment, while it is day 8-10 gave a similar treatment as before but now got all participants placebo capsules along with the drink. Vid day 1, day 3, day 8 and day 10 were taken blood samples of participants for analysis of the immune system's response to treatment.

The researchers found that, for the first time managed to show a conditioned reflex in the human immune system where it is with a specially designed beverage linked to a regular treatment with immunosuppressive drugs could have a view that man with the special potion (placebo) then of the person been able to obtain almost the same immune reduction effect that the medicinal product in this case cyclosporine A give. Professor Schedlowski believes that this research will be able to bring to you in a future with method conditioned reflex, to reduce the need of drugs at transplantation. This gives less side effects and lower costs for the lifelong treatment. The method can probably also be used at other auto-immune diseases such as Rheumatoid artrit or psoriasis. Further research will, among other things examine the mechanism behind that some people respond very well to the conditioned treatment with placebo while others have smaller effects of the treatment. Possibly, genetic factors are in mixed in different people's response to conditioned placebo.

Other studies have also shown that if a patient regularly taken medicine aspirin where it was marked by the pills shape, color and taste and replaces the treatment with inactive placebo pills with similar performance as the patient may feel pain relief via placebo effect. Generally it can be said that the placebo treatment after an earlier drug-treatment has major effect than if the placebo is given for the first time, showing on a learning effect. Experiments have shown that there is a correlation between the placebo pills shape by capsules has greater impact than pills and tablets color can affect to varying degrees depending of the treated the disease. The following colors has proven to work best during research.

Yellow tablets   -effectiveness against depression

Red tablets   -stimulant, awakening effect

Green tablets   -anxiety dampening

Blue tablets   -calming effect

White tablets   -antidepressant effect, even at such as peptic ulcer.

Placebo has also the existence of a hierarchy of placebo treatment there increasing effect is given by the following order: tablets, capsules, injections, acupuncture or fake surgery interventions. In general, the placebo showed a greater impact on psychological disease states or psychosomatic diseases, while in the case of, for example cancer or viral diseases have not been able to document any significant impact.

Experiences of how doctors and paramedics responding to patients have also been shown in research to greatly affect the patient's pain experience and the influence of placebo/nocebo effects. It is important that the patient becomes "seen" and taken on seriously and that the verbal information from the doctor is extremely central. Information on potential side effects of drugs or treatments should be given on a way so that the nocebo effects are minimized. The research in the placebo effect is focused on to understand the mechanisms of the brain behind for example pain relief and in the future be able to maximize the positive contributions of placebo effect in the treatment of various medical conditions. As mentioned in Chapter 8 of hypnosis, from a historical point of view, pointed out how for example Axel Munthe in his book "the book of San Michele" also touches on the subject of placebo. In several chapters outlines he for how to provide diagnoses of different welfare symptoms in their often female upper-class patients with fabricated diagnoses such as Appendicitis or Colitis. This has led to obvious placebo effects and, of course, a good regular income. This type of treatment resulted in a tying of the patient to the doctor for prolonged treatments.

As we have seen in the chapters on biofeedback, hypnosis and placebo, pain-conditions are affected by different types of treatments. In the case of psychosomatic illnesses have on later time also CBT (cognitive behavioral therapy) and other psychological therapies have been shown to have similar effect that treatment with placebo give, among others treatment of disease IBS (Irritable Bowel Syndrome). Earlier has it not known if it is the same mechanism that is behind the analgesic effect of these different treatments, but with fMRI, PET and MEG have a more accurate mapping of the different brain areas involved in pain experiences have been carried out. In a study "Brain activity during pain relief using hypnosis and placebo treatments: A literature review" (see ref. 9.15) is Svetlana Kirjanen at the University of Helsinki, Finland made a comparative literature study on the mechanisms behind hypnosis and placebo. The study result in that it is some common mechanisms between hypnosis and the placebo treatment, but also differences which show that there are different areas of the brain's total pain network affected depending of the selected treatment method (see table 9.1)

Table 9.1 Pain impact

Brain area	Hypnosis	Placebo
Somatosensory cortex	X	X
Insula	X	X
Thalamus	X	X
ACC	X	X
Prefrontal cortex	X	X
Amygdala		X
Hypothalamus		X
Hippocampus		X
PAG		X
Nucleus accumbens		X
Occipital cortex	X	
Basal ganglia	X	

Research in the placebo is affecting much of the detail processes with neurochemical while hypnosis research is directed towards clinical research and if it involves different States of consciousness. Research on the interaction between "Body/Mind" is interesting and should be multidisciplinary, as mechanisms of biofeedback, hypnosis, placebo and psychological therapies probably has more common basics.

Cultural conditioned placebo

Homeopathy is an alternative medicine school, where one may surmise that placebo effect often is the only curative effect. Homeopathy is based on theories from the doctor Samuel Hanemann (1755-1843) in which the basic idea is that a substance that can cause certain pathological symptoms in a healthy individual can cure the same symptoms in a sick person. The principle is called "similars" or "Similia Similibus curentur" and emanates from then on 1790 Hanemann century experimented with quinine bark that at times was used for treatment of chills at malaria and discovered that if he took a low dose of the drug had the same symptoms as malaria illness suffered as lightheadedness, chills and skeleton pain. This principle "similars" derives, among other things from Paracelsus (1493-1541) which in his writing 250 years earlier expressed this principle. This "discovery" led to Hanemann continued a systematic exploration of that test herbs and minerals in healthy people and see what effect they gave and then treat patients who have these symptoms with "medicinal product". Until about 1800 had Hanemann systematically tried out about 90 different organic and inorganic substances under this system and started using them in his medical practice.

In 1810 he published Hanemann, the book "Organen der Rationellen Heilkunde" which then was the starting point for further development of homeopathy. Today includes a revised version "Materia Medica" about 2,000 homeopathic remedies. Homeopathy claims also that a "drug" becomes more potent the more substance is diluted out in for example water. It says that the dilution releases dynamic forces that exist in the healing substance. There are three different system to manufacture homeopathic medicines where the letters D = 10 times, C = 100 times and LM = 50000 times specifies the factor between each level of dilution, for example. D2 = 100 times, C2 = 10000 times, D6 = 1 million times, D9 = 1 billion times and at D23 has Avogadro's number achieved which says that most likely there is no matter of the drug left. In addition, the bottle at each dilution is struck against a hard object a prescribed number of times to release healing power.

Theory about potent is that the effect of a drug is inversely proportional to its active substance and power in a topic is in the pattern and the less of the substance the greater the force. It is explained by some form of energy are formed and strengthened by solution shaken rhythmically at the dilutions. According to homeopathy by "equally curable with equally" involved subjects who develop symptoms of the disease to the body's immune system is activated. It also says that every disease is individual and, therefore, it is not certain that the same medicines should be used with two different people with the same symptoms. Homeopathy emphasizes that we must treat the entire body and that it just is the sick cells that react to printed homeopathic medicine.

The previous audit of the current placebo research in this chapter indicates that placebo effects can be obtained and is affected by many different mechanisms in a patient's brain functions and external influences from the surrounding environment. The incredible dilution of active substances in homeopathic medicinal products, with great probability is excluded as it works-the same part in a homeopathic treatment. On the other hand , the usually positive and in depth talks on the patient's medical image and symptoms, which may include a two-hour visit, contribute to a placebo effect according to the previously described research. Placebo effect is amplified by the prescription of one or several homeopathic medicinal products with a positive verbal suggestion about its healing effect. Some homeopaths have even electronic measuring equipment that can reinforce placebo effects.

In the course of human history, are diseases and afflictions through epidemics ravaged with much suffering and death. Before the later part of 1800 century began to take up active medications and introduce hygienic conditions was to extradited to the doctor, medicine men or "Wise men/women" that did not have access to medications such as antibiotics without used cupping and bloodletting as a panacea. These cures could in many contexts result in deterioration of the patient's general condition for serious disease. The active component in the treatments was the patient's capacity for self-healing, which supported of placebo effect from the often charismatic doctors/medicine men and their decocted.

A modern variant of this activity is likely to be strong depending of placebo effect is in , among other things the charismatic Christian revival, where healers through the laying on of hands and prayer heals people through in with faith help. Especially in the United States seem a number of pastors in TV-broadcast meetings where we for example could see Peter Popoff in a three hour faith-healing church service scream and ranting in God's name. It arranged a queue of suffering at the stage edge where the healer takes care of them one by one. Through the laying on of hands and the ousting of evil spirits detached from Satan and many collapse on the floor of the movement in the inflated mood is often accompanied by evocative music. Miracle is illustrated by that I'll throw crutches and go or traveling up from the wheelchair and to speak to about that bones have been extended during healing. The magician James Randi, collaborating with organization CSI (Committee for Skeptical Inquiry) which examines alleged supernatural phenomena, have out-feel like a reward of $ 1 million to anyone who can prove some kind of supernatural phenomena and examined the phenomenon of faith-healing in the 1980 's. Randi reviewed the TV-felt healer Popoffs methods during the 1985-1986 and could, among other things reveal a secret radio communications between Popoffs wife Elizabeth and Popoff in where information collected about the visitors before the meeting were used as inspirations from God. Also for example method that back problems depending on alleged differences in a visitor's leg length should be addressed through healing, appeared to be manipulated with the proper camera angles and the manipulation of one shoe's location on foot. In TV program devoted much time to affect viewers to donate money to the organization that supported the Popoff. Randi's revealing got great attention in the United States and resulted in bankruptcy for Popoffs organization, in 1987.

If you today are looking for on the internet are the same type of activity started again and Peter Popoff sells through its TV programs (which are broadcast over TV networks both in the United States, Europe and Australia) "Miracle Spring Water", "Holy Sand" and "Miracle Manna". These products have miraculous effects and provide both bot for disease and affect the success of such as economic affairs. As we've seen on research regarding placebo, the charismatic effect of a spiritual healer (faith healers) probably affect psychosomatic diseases, but it is fallacious to claim these miracle, with great financial gain, regarding for example leg extension and to give cancer patients false for reflections about the cure. The effect is instead placebo effects of endorphins and maybe dopamine with short-term pain relief. The healer also claims often that if one doesn't get healed, it is because the belief in God is not strong enough, which may put the person in mental crisis.

Even in Sweden have faith-healing recently examined in the program "Cold Facts" on TV4, where the healer Jens Garnfeldt from Denmark who operations in several countries, i.e. Sweden has been reviewed. In the program shows that use Garnfeldt similar methods with leg extension and promised by the bot of cancer as in the American model and invites visitors to give great gifts to the organization behind Garnfeldt. During a meeting claiming Garnfeldt i.e. that God said to him that there are a number of people in the room who can provide totals on 10000 crowns each. This type of manipulation often affects older people to take off their already low income in order to give away its last money. Many local congregations in the Swedish Evangelical Alliance (SEA) dismiss these independent preachers and their activities.

In historical perspective, see in the most primitive tribes on Earth all continents different forms of belief in elemental beings (such as animism, shamanism) and on the deceased the ancestral spirit. Different priest, medicine men, shamans or nåjder has via legends, rituals and often in trance during ecstatic trance conveyed messages from the spirit world. But they are also contracted for the cure of diseases through healing or making decoctions of herbs or talismans as loaded with special magical power. One of these religions is Voodoo religion that is practiced in many forms for example Haiti, Puerto Rico, New Orleans in the United States and West Africa. In voodoo rites are part of the worship of the ancestors and spirits that are a kind of animistic religions. In Haiti's voodoo people religion along with Roman Catholicism. There are some drifts sometimes voodoo religions in which it can be part of the rites that shape the zombies, which is a person who by poison been deprived of his free will. The creation of zombies has been used in some quarters as cheap labor and creation of zombies are attributed to mighty houngans (voodoo priests) who have access to complex toxins and ceremonies for the creation of a zombie. Another perversion is the creation of voodoo dolls (to be emulating current person) in which the man sticking needles and pronounce curses to using black magic to affect the person negatively or even requests for the life out of him.

In this type of tribal societies can it through to the designated person is excluded from the community and is treated bad lead to one for early death depending of the mental stress that the person subjected to lecturer. We can say that in such a case of the nocebo effect can the idea of the curse and the belief in voodoo priest affect the autonomic nervous system that cause disease or to and with death. Possible that it is placebo positive items involved in the curative effects of diseases.

In this chapter that highlighted research on the placebo/nocebo effects shows that later time new methods with fMRI, MEG, PET and EEG equipment has been able to provide completely new understanding of the different centers in the brain that are involved in pain perception. Among other things, the importance of the body's own endorphins and the neurotransmitter dopamine has been shown to reduce pain even with a placebo pill (sugar pill). Future research is focused on in ordinary medical treatment safeguard placebo to find synergies to maximize effect of medications and treatments of medical conditions. An interesting aspect is that the previous related pain treatments such as biofeedback, hypnosis, and placebo have similar effect as CBT and other psychological therapies on psychosomatic diseases and should be studied for different disciplines to identify basic common mechanisms in the brain.

After writing

This book is the result of two years of intense study of the accelerating results from the current brain research. Among other things, the ongoing project "The human connectome" project in the United States and "Human Brain project" in Europe generates new knowledge in fast pace. In my 34 years with research and development of radar systems for Fighter aircraft Viggen and the JAS project, I have encountered many colleagues with similar experience of implicit learning (tacit knowledge) which is conveyed in the book. This suggests on that we have a hidden capacity in the brain which unconsciously is involved when we are faced with new harder problem tasks. One can hope that the new scientific findings will help us find ways to support these unconscious processes in the brain.

For inspiration for the book, I am grateful for all the discussions around the coffee table on EMW, where many of these issues have been raised by my colleague. Special thanks are due to the two managers who hired me at EMW and which served as my mentors. Rune Jackobsson (Jack) was my first Group Manager and was who that has shaped my view on logic and science knowledge. Moreover Ingvar Sundström, later on head of the whole JAS radar development worked as my mentor with brilliant technical leadership.

In the section about Aikido would I thank Ulf Evenås (7th Dan) for access to video material. In addition, have discussions with members in Göteborgs Aikido Dojo has brought new knowledge. Special thanks goes to the Aikido members Ronny Irekvist (6 Dan) and Zeth Moberg (6 Dan) for their in-depth discussions.

When it comes to the design of the neurological section of the book is a special thanks to Rolf Ekman professor emeritus in neurochemistry at the Göteborgs University and Per-Olof Nilsson, professor emeritus of physics at Chalmers University of Technology for good advice and inspiration. Finally, thanks to my partner Lena as a support and a sounding board for the book's creation. Lena has also designed the graphic design of the book's insertion and book covers.

REFERENCES
Chapter 1

1.1 Aurelius Augustinus, år 397, (bok11, § 17-41): *Confessions and enchiridion*, translation: Albert C Outler.

1.2 M.S. Gazzaniga, I.E. Bogen, R.W. Sperry, 1963: *Laterality effects in some thesis following cerebral commissurotomy in man.*

1.3 M.S. Gazzaniga, I.E. Bogen, R.W. Sperry, 1965: *Observations on visual perception after disconnexion of the cerebral hemispheres in man.*

1.4 D. O. Hebb, 1949, Organization of behaviour: *A neuropsychological theory.* New York: John Wiley and Sons.

1.5 H. Georg Kuhn et al., 2009: Cardiovascular fitness is associated with cognition in young adulthood. PNAS volym 106 no. 49.

1.6 Hans Berger, 1929: *Über das Elektroenzephalogramm des Menschen. Archiv für Psychiatrie und Nervenkrankheiten*, 1929, 87: 527-570.

1.7 Hans H. Kornhuber, Lyder Deecke, 1965: *Hirnpotentialänderungen bei willkyrbewegungen und passiven Bewegungen des Mensch: Bereitschaftspotential und reafferente potentiale.*

1.8 Libet et al., 1964: *Production of threshold levels of conscious sensation by electrical stimulation of human somatosensory cortex*, Journal of Neurophysiology 27.

1.9 Libet et al. 1967: *Responses of human somatosensory cortex to stimuli below threshold for conscious sensation*, Science 158.

1.10 Libet et al., 1979: *Subjective Referral of the Timing for a Conscious Sensory Experience*, Brain 102.

1.11 Libet et al. 1983: *Time of conscious intention to act in relation to onset of cerebral activity (readiness potential): the unconscious initiation of a freely voluntary act*, Brain 106.

1.12 Libet et al., 1991: *Control of the transition from sensory detection to sensory awareness in man by the duration of thalamic stimulus. The cerebral "time-on" factor*, Brain 114.

1.13 David Chalmers, 1995: *Facing up to the problem of consciousness*, Journal of consciousness studies 2.

1.14 Libet, 1994, *A testable field theory of mind-brain interaction*, JCS 1.

1.15 Wolf Singer, 2007, *Binding by synchrony*, Scholarpedia 2.

1.16 John-Dylan Haynes et al., 2011, *tracking the unconscious generation of free decisions using ultra-high field fMRI*, DOI 10.1371/journal. pone.0021612.

1.17 Marcus Raichle, Debra Gusnard, 2001, *searching for a baseline: Functional imaging and the resting human brain*. Nature Reviews Neuroscience, vol.2.

1.18 Martijn van den Heuvel, Olaf Sporns, 2011, *Rich-Club Organization of Human Connectome*, Journal of Neuroscience.

1.19 Martijn van den Heuvel, Olaf Sporns, et al. 2013, *Abnormal Rich Club Organization and Functional Brain Dynamics in Schizophrenia*, JAMA Psychiatry vol. 70.

Litterature

Christoph Fahlke et al., 2012, *Fysiologisk bildordbok*, Liber AB.

Lars Olson, Anna Josephson (red.), 2012, *Hjärnan*, Karolinska Institutet University Press.

Tor Nörrestranders, 1999, *Märk världen - en bok om vetenskap och intuition*, Bonnier Alba.

Chapter 2

2.1 Christof Koch, 2004, *The Quest for consciousness*, Roberts & company publishers.

2.2 Ungerleider L. G., Mishkin M,1982, *Two cortical system, Analysis of visual behaviour*, MIT press

2.3 Marco Tamietto, Beatrice de Gelder et al., 2009, *Unseen facial bodily expressions trigger fast emotional reactions*, PNA, vol. 106, No 42.

2.4 Lucy Donaldson, Jan Melichar, 2007, *A taste of depression*, University of Bristol Research review, Issue 14, april 2007.

2.5 Devin Terhune et al., 2011, *Enhanced Cortical Excitability in Grapheme-Color Synesthesia and its Modulation*, Current Biology 21, december 2011.

2.6 D Brang et al., 2010, *Magnetoencephalography revels early activation of V4 in grapheme-color synesthesia,* Neuroimage 53.

2.7 Allan W Snyder et al., 2011, *Facilitate Insight by Non-Invasive Brain Stimulation*, PLos ONE, Volume 6, Issue2.

Litterature

Jan Ygge, 2011, *Ögat och synen,* University press.

Chapter 3

3.1 L Gallant et al., 2009, *Bayesian Reconstruction of Natural Images from Human Brain Activity,* Neuron 63.

3.2 L Gallant, 2011, *Reconstruction Visual Experiences from Brain Activity Evoked by Natural Movies*, Current Biology 21.

3.3 Y Kamitoni et al., 2013, *Neutral Decoding of Visual Imagery During Sleep*, Science Vol. 340.

3.4 Demis Hassabis et al, 2009, *Decoding Neuronal Ensembles in Human Hippocampus,* Current Biology 19.

3.5 Haynes et al., 2007, *Reading Hidden Intentions in the Human Brain,* Current Biology 17.

3.6 Owen AM et al, 2010, *Willful modulation of brain activity in disorders of consciousness,* The new England Journal of Medicine, 362

3.7 Gerwin Schalk et al, 2012, *Decoding onset and direction of movements using Electrocorticographic (ECoG) signals in humans*, Frontiers in neuroengineering, vol. 5

3.8 Brunner P et al, 2015, *Brain-to-text: Decoding spoken sentences from phone representations in the brain,* journal of Frontiers in neuroengineering, Doi. 10.3389/fnins.2015.00217

3.9 Picard R W et al, 2006, *Self-Cam Feedback From What Would be your Social Partner,* Research Posters, Boston MA august 3 page 138

3.10 Andy Mckinley et al, 2013, *Acceleration of image Analyst Training with Transcranial Direct Current Stimulation*, Wright State Research Institute Publications

3.11 Läkartidningen, 2009, nummer 14, *Vbait Liest has treated 300 patients with TMS.*

3.12 Rajesh Rao, 2014, *A direct Brain-to-Brain Interface in Humans*, PLOS Doi: 10.1371/journal.pone.0111332

Chapter 4

4.1 Baris Sentuna, G Babayigit Irez, et al. *Six months aikido training shortens reaction time*, International journal of Human Sciences, se ref. 4

4.2 S. Stenudd, 1995, *Fem ringars bok, Rin no Sho*, Arriba förlag

4.3 Morihei Ueshiba, 2002, *The art of peace*. Shambhala

Litterature

Stefan Stenudd, 1998, *Aikido- den fredliga kampkonsten*, Arriba förlag

Stefan Stenudd et al. 2010, *Tävling, träning, tradition Svensk budo och kampsport 50 år*, Arriba förlag

John Stevens, 1989, *The sword of no-sword, Life of the master warrior Tesshu, Shambhala*

Zeth Moberg, 2001, *Den pastellblå hunden*, Prius Press

Chapter 5

5.1 K Stanovich, J Evans, 2013, *Dual-process theories of higher cognition: Advancing the debate*,

5.2 Daniel Kahneman, 2013, Think fast and slow,Bokförlag Volante

5.3 D Kahneman, 1974, A Tversky, *Judgment under uncertainty: Heuristics and biases*, Science, Vol. 185 No 407

5.4 Klein, 1988, *Rapid Decision Making on the fire ground*, Technical report 796, 1988, U. S. Army

5.5 Kahneman, 2009, *Conditions for intuitive expertise: a failure to disagree*, American Psychologist, Vol. 64 No 6

5.6 Praesto, 1997, Intuition: En bok om hur du utnyttjar dina dolda resurser, Liber AB

Chapter 6

6.1 G. Rizzolatti et al., 1996, *Action recognition in the premotor cortex*, Brain 119, 593-609

6.2 Julius Fast, 1970, *Body language*, Simon & Schulster Adult Publishing group

6.3 Amy Cuddy, 2010, *Power Posing, Brief Nonverbal dispalays Affect Neuroendocrine Levels and Risk Tolerance,*Psychological Science 21

6.4 William James, 1890, *Principles of Psychology*

Kapitel 7

7.1 Barbara Brown, 1982, *Psyches hidden power,* Wahlström & Widstrand

7.2 Chase, M.H., Sterman, M.B., 1967, *Maturation of patterns of sleep and wakefulness in the kitten.* Brain Research, 5:319-329

7.3 Sterman M.B., McDonald L.R., 1978, *Effects of central cortical EEG feedback training on incidence of poorly controlled seizures.* Epilepsia, 19(3):207-222

7.4 Christopher deCharms et al., 2005, *Control over brain activation and pain learned by using real-time functional* MRI, PNA Vol. 102 no 51

7.5 Lawrence A. Farwell et al., 2013, *Brain fingerprinting field studies comparing P300-MERMER and P300 brainwave responses in the detection of concealed information,* Cognitive Neurodynamics, Vol. 7, Issue 14

7.6 Chris Berker et al., 2010, *Accelerating Training Using Interactive Neuro- Educational Technologies: Applications to Archery, Golf and Rifle Marksmanship,* The International Journal of sport & society, Vol 1

Chapter 8

8.1 David Spiegel et al, 2012, *Functional Brain Basis of Hypnotizability,* Archives of General Psychiatry, vol. 69 no 10

8.2 John Hartland, 1974, *Klinisk hypnos,* Natur och kultur

8.3 F Roelants, C Watremez et al, 2011, *Breast cancer surgery under hypnosis and local anaesthesia: Feasibility and potential benefits:* 8AP5-8, Vol. 28

8.4 F.L. Marcuse, 1960, *Hypnos,* Prisma

8.5 S Kallio et al, 2011, *The existence of Hypnotic State Revealed by Eye Movements*, PLOS ONE/6(10):e 26374 doi:10.1371/journal.pone 0026374

8.6 S Kallio, 2013, *A Preconscious Neural Mechanism of Hypnotically Altered Colors: A Double Case Study*, PLOS One8(8):e 70900 doi:10.1371/lournal.pone.007900

Chapter 9

9.1 Beecher H K, 1955, *The powerful placebo*, Journal Am. Med. Association, 159 (17):1602-6

9.2 F Benedetti, 2008, *Placebo Effects: Understanding the mechanisms in health and disease*, Oxford Press

9.3 F Benedetti, 2011, *the many placebo effects*, Spanda Journal 11.1

9.4 I Kirsch et al, 1998, *Listening to Prozac but hearing placebo: a metaanalysis of antidepressant medication*, Prevention & Treatment, Vol. 1(2)

9.5 I Kirsch, 2010, *The emperor`s new drugs: Exploring the antidepressing myth*, Basic Books

9.6 P Petrovic, 2005, *Placebo in emotional processing-induced expectations of anxiety relief activate a generalized modulatory network*, Neuro 46, 957-969

9.7 P Petrovic et al, 2002, *Placebo and opioid analgesia-imaging a shard neuronal network*, Science 295, 1737-1740

9.8 F Eippert et al, 2009, *Activation of opioidergic descending pain control systems underlines placebo analgesia,* Neuron 63, 533-543

9.9 F Benedetti, 2008, *The role of learning in placebo and placebo effects*, Pain 136, 211-218

9.10 F Benedetti et al, 1997, *Blockade of nocebo hyperalgesia by the cholecystokinin antagonist proglumide*, Pain 71, 135-140

9.11 F Benedetti et al, 2006, *The biochemical and neuroendocrine bases of the hyperalgesic nocebo effect*, J. Neurosci 26, 12014–12022

9.12 David J Scott et al, 2007, *Individual Differences in Reward Responding Explain Placebo-Induced Expectations and effects*, Neuron 55, 325-336

9.13 Martin Ingvar et al, 2012, *Nonconscious activation of placebo and nocebo pain response,* Vol. 109, no 39, 15959-15964, doi: 10.1073/pnas.1202056109

9.14 M Schedlowski, et al, 2002, *Behavioural conditioning of immunosuppression is possible in humans*, the FASEB journal vol. 16 no 14, 1869-1873

9.15 Svetlana Kirjanen, 2011, *the brain activity during pain relief using hypnosis and placebo treatments: A literature review*, efpsa Vol.3 no 1